ADVANCES IN
Vascular Surgery

VOLUME 6

ADVANCES IN
Vascular Surgery

VOLUME 1

VOLUME 4

ADVANCES IN

Vascular Surgery

VOLUME 6

Editor-in-Chief
Anthony D. Whittemore, M.D.
Professor of Surgery, Harvard University Medical School; Chief, Division of Vascular Surgery, Brigham and Women's Hospital, Boston, Massachusetts

Associate Editors
Dennis F. Bandyk, M.D.
Professor of Surgery, University of South Florida College of Medicine; Director, Vascular Surgery Division, Tampa, Florida

Jack L. Cronenwett, M.D.
Professor of Surgery, Dartmouth Medical School; Chief, Section of Vascular Surgery, Dartmouth–Hitchcock Medical Center, Lebanon, New Hampshire

Norman R. Hertzer, M.D.
Chairman, Department of Vascular Surgery, Cleveland Clinic Foundation, Cleveland, Ohio

Rodney A. White, M.D.
Professor of Surgery, University of California at Los Angeles School of Medicine; Chief of Vascular Surgery, Associate Chairman, Department of Surgery, Harbor–University of California at Los Angeles Medical Center, Torrance, California

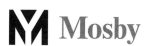 Mosby

St. Louis   Baltimore   Boston   Carlsbad   Naples   New York   Philadelphia   Portland
London   Madrid   Mexico City   Singapore   Sydney   Tokyo   Toronto   Wiesbaden

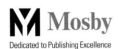

Mosby

Dedicated to Publishing Excellence

A Times Mirror
Company

Publisher: Theresa Van Schaik
Developmental Editor: Sarah Zagarri
Manager, Periodical Editing: Kirk Swearingen
Production Editor: Amanda Maguire
Project Supervisor, Production: Joy Moore
Production Assistant: Laura Bayless

Printed in the United States of America
Composition by The Clarinda Company
Printing/binding by The Maple-Vail Book Manufacturing Company

Mosby, Inc.
11830 Westline Industrial Drive
St. Louis, Missouri 63146

International Standard Serial Number: 1069–7292
International Standard Book Number: 0–8151–8415–8

Contributors

Peter Bell, M.D., F.R.C.S.
Professor of Surgery, University of Leicester, Leicester, England

John J. Bergan, M.D., F.A.C.S., F.R.C.S. (Hon.), Eng.
Clinical Professor of Surgery, University of California, San Diego; Professor of Surgery, Loma Linda University Medical Center, Loma Linda, California; Clinical Professor of Surgery, Uniformed Services University of the Health Sciences, Bethesda, Maryland; Professor of Surgery Emeritus, Northwestern University Medical School, Chicago, Illinois

Amman Bolia, M.B.Ch.B., F.R.C.S.
Consultant Vascular Radiologist, Leicester Royal Infirmary, Leicester, England

David C. Brewster, M.D.
Clinical Professor of Surgery, Massachusetts General Hospital and Harvard Medical School, Boston, Massachusetts

Nancy L. Cantelmo, M.D.
Associate Professor of Surgery, Boston University School of Medicine; Associate Chief of Surgery, Boston Veterans Administration Medical Center, Boston, Massachusetts

Jae-Sung Cho, M.D.
Fellow, Division of Vascular Surgery, Mayo Clinic, Rochester, Minnesota

G. Patrick Clagett, M.D.
Pickens Professor of Medical Science; Chief, Division of Vascular Surgery, University of Texas Southwestern Medical Center, Dallas, Texas

John E. Connolly, D.P.M.
Assistant Professor of Surgery (Podiatry), Dartmouth Medical School, Hanover, New Hampshire; Staff Podiatrist and Director, Podiatric Medical Education, Veterans Affairs Medical Center, White River Junction, Vermont

Michael S. Conte, M.D.
Assistant Professor of Surgery, Harvard Medical School, Attending Surgeon, Department of Surgery and Section of Vascular Surgery, Brigham and Women's Hospital, Boston, Massachusetts

James M. Cooper, M.D.
Assistant Professor of Radiology, Mount Sinai School of Medicine, Attending Radiologist, The Mount Sinai Medical Center, New York, New York

Thomas J. Fogarty, M.D.
Professor of Surgery, Stanford University Medical Center, Stanford, California

Peter Gloviczki, M.D.
Professor of Surgery, Mayo Medical School; Vice Chair, Division of Vascular Surgery, Mayo Clinic, Rochester, Minnesota

Thomas M. Grist, M.D.
Associate Professor, Department of Radiology, University of Wisconsin Hospital and Clinics, Madison, Wisconsin

Ryan T. Hagino, M.D.
Assistant Professor of Surgery, University of Texas Health Science Center at San Antonio; Attending Staff, Wilford Hall Medical Center, Lackland AFB, Texas

Kimberley J. Hansen, M.D.
Associate Professor of Surgery, Department of General Surgery, Wake Forest University School of Medicine, Winston-Salem, North Carolina

George D. Hermann, B.S.M.E.
General Manager, Fogarty Research, Portola Valley, California

Larry H. Hollier, M.D.
Julius H. Jacobson II, M.D., Professor of Vascular Surgery, Chairman, Department of Surgery, Mount Sinai School of Medicine, Surgeon in Chief, The Mount Sinai Medical Center, New York, New York

Michael J. Mann, M.D.
Instructor of Cardiovascular Medicine, Harvard Medical School, Associate Physician, Brigham and Women's Hospital, Boston, Massachusetts

Michael L. Marin, M.D.
Associate Professor of Surgery, Mount Sinai School of Medicine, Director, Endovascular Surgical Development, The Mount Sinai Medical Center, New York, New York

James May, M.S., F.R.A.C.S., F.A.C.S.
Bosch Professor of Surgery, Department of Surgery, University of Sydney; Attending Surgeon, Department of Vascular Surgery, Royal Prince Alfred Hospital, Sydney, New South Wales, Australia

Martha D. McDaniel, M.D.
Associate Professor of Surgery, Dartmouth Medical School, Hanover, New Hampshire; Acting Chief, Surgical Service, Veterans Affairs Medical Center, White River Junction, Vermont

Harold A. Mitty, M.D.
Professor of Radiology, Mount Sinai School of Medicine, Attending Radiologist, The Mount Sinai Medical Center, New York, New York

Timothy C. Oskin, M.D.
Vascular Surgery Fellow, Department of General Surgery, Wake Forest University School of Medicine, Winston-Salem, North Carolina

Richard Parsons, M.D.
Assistant Professor of Surgery, Mount Sinai School of Medicine, The Mount Sinai Medical Center, New York, New York

Julian J. Pribaz, M.D.
Associate Professor of Surgery, Harvard Medical School, Brigham and Women's Hospital, Boston, Massachusetts

Kim M. Rozokat, C.O.T.A.
Certified Occupational Therapy Assistant, Veterans Affairs Medical Center, White River Junction, Vermont

Christian E. Sampson, M.D.
Instructor in Surgery, Harvard Medical School, Brigham and Women's Hospital, Boston, Massachusetts

Eugene D. Strandness, Jr., M.D.
Professor, Department of Surgery, University of Washington School of Medicine, Seattle, Washington

Gerald R. Sydorak, M.D.
Clinical Associate Professor of Surgery, University of California at San Francisco, San Francisco, California; Staff Vascular Surgeon, Mills Peninsula Hospital, Burlingame, California

Roy L. Tawes, M.D.
Chief of Surgery, Mills Peninsula Hospital, Burlingame, California; Clinical Professor of Surgery, University of California at San Francisco, San Francisco, California

William D. Turnipseed, M.D.
Professor, Department of Surgery, Section of Vascular Surgery, University of Wisconsin Hospital and Clinics, Madison, Wisconsin

Daniel B. Walsh, M.D.
Professor of Surgery, Section of Vascular Surgery, Dartmouth-Hitchcock Medical Center, Lebanon, New Hampshire

L. Albert Wetter, M.D.
Mills Peninsula Hospital, Burlingame, California; Instructor in Surgery, University of California at San Francisco, San Francisco, California

Geoffrey H. White, M.B., B.S.
Clinical Associate Professor of Surgery, Department of Surgery, University of Sydney; Attending Surgeon, Department of Vascular Surgery, Royal Prince Alfred Hospital, Sydney, New South Wales, Australia

James S. Wrobel, M.S., D.P.M.
Adjunct Assistant Professor, Departments of Family and Community Medicine and Surgery (Podiatry), Dartmouth Medical School, Hanover, New Hampshire; Staff Podiatrist, Veterans Affairs Medical Center, White River Junction, Vermont

Contents

PART III Venous Disease

6. Evolution of Varicose Vein Surgery
By John J. Bergan, M.D., F.A.C.S., F.R.C.S. (Hon.), Eng. 81

7. Balloon Dissection for Endoscopic Subfascial Ligation
By Roy L Tawes, L. Albert Wetter, Gerald R. Sydorak,
George D. Hermann, and Thomas J. Fogarty 93

8. Renal Revascularization for Salvage: Results of Treatment for Renal Artery Occlusion
By Kimberley J. Hansen and Timothy C. Oskin 103

PART I

Carotid Artery Disease

CHAPTER 1

Impact of Plaque Morphology in Carotid Disease

Nancy L. Cantelmo, M.D.
Associate Professor of Surgery, Boston University School of Medicine;
Associate Chief of Surgery, Boston Veterans Administration Medical
Center, Boston, Massachusetts

It is well established that the degree of internal carotid artery (ICA) stenosis is the most important criterion in the selection of patients as candidates for carotid endarterectomy (CEA). The North American Symptomatic Carotid Endarterectomy Trial (NASCET) reported that surgery was the optimal treatment for patients with symptomatic ICA stenosis of greater than 70% when compared with medical management.[1] The Asymptomatic Carotid Atherosclerosis Study (ACAS) concluded that surgery was better than medical therapy for stoke prevention in patients with greater than 60% ICA stenosis who had no symptoms of transient ischemic attack (TIA) or stroke.[2] Many questions still unanswered relate to other categories of patients with carotid artery disease who might best be managed by surgery to prevent cerebral infarction.

Attention has been focused on various aspects of plaque morphology in an effort to understand its relationship to stroke risk. The composition and surface characteristics of carotid artery plaque have been the subject of many investigations, which have studied both the methods of detection and the clinical significance of plaque morphology.

This chapter will review some of the work reported in the literature concerning plaque morphology. The author will offer a perspective on management of patients with regard to the various aspects of plaque form and structure based on our current understanding of the subject.

1

INTRAPLAQUE HEMORRHAGE

For many years vascular surgeons have noted intraplaque hemorrhage (IPH) as a characteristic of the carotid artery plaque encountered during CEA. Many investigators have demonstrated a correlation between symptoms of TIA and stroke and IPH.[3] In an often quoted study by Imperato and co-workers[4] who examined 376 CEA specimens, IPH was the only plaque characteristic found more commonly in the specimens of symptomatic patients when compared with those of asymptomatic patients.

According to their study, these observations were only applicable to patients with an ICA stenosis greater than 70%. These results were corroborated by Lusby.[5] He and his co-workers studied neurologic symptoms not only in relationship to the occurrence of IPH, but also with regard to the histologically determined age of the IPH. Neurologic symptoms correlated better with more acute hemorrhage than older hemorrhage.

With the development of duplex ultrasound, many researchers reported that IPH could be accurately identified using this modality when compared with actual plaque specimens from CEA. In addition to identifying the presence of IPH, ultrasound is able to provide information on the relative quantity of hemorrhage as well as its location with regard to the luminal surface of the artery. Some investigators have suggested that a larger relative quantity of IPH and a location closer to the luminal surface may be more significant.

PLAQUE CHARACTERIZATION

Further studies with duplex ultrasound have led to the characterization of carotid plaque as either homogeneous or heterogeneous. Homogeneous plaque is sonographically uniform with low-level echoes, and is designated as echogenic.

It most often has a smooth surface. When this type of plaque is examined histologically, it is found to be composed of dense, fibrous connective tissue. Heterogeneous plaque is complex and demonstrates at least one focal echolucent area within the plaque. These lucent areas correlate to IPH.

In an attempt to further clarify plaque characteristics, a classification system was proposed by Gray-Weale and co-workers.[6] In their scheme, a Type 1 lesion is mainly echolucent, often with a thin echogenic cap; Type 2 is mostly echolucent with small areas of echogenicity; Type 3 lesions are mostly echogenic with less than 25% area of echolucency; and Type 4 lesions are uniformly echogenic. Types 1 and 2 correspond to heterogeneous plaque, thought to contain areas of IPH, whereas Types 3 and 4 correlate with homogeneous plaque of a predominantly fibrous nature.

Heterogeneity of carotid plaque has also been associated with neurologic symptoms by a number of investigators.[3] In a prospective study by Sterpetti et al.,[7] it was shown that heterogeneous plaque was a risk factor for development of symptoms in a group of patients followed for a year. These authors also reported that plaque heterogeneity and degree of ICA stenosis were independent variables with respect to symptoms.

Geroulakos and co-workers[8] showed that the more echolucent Types 1 and 2 plaques were found more often in symptomatic patients, and the predominantly echogenic Types 3 and 4 plaques in those patients without symptoms. These findings proved valid only in those patients with greater than 70% stenosis. This group also demonstrated a significantly greater number of cerebral infarctions by CT in patients with a stenosis of greater than 70% and Type 1 plaque than in all other patient groups combined.

In a study of the natural history of asymptomatic plaques, Bock and colleagues[9] identified a 5.7% annual rate of TIA and stroke in patients with echolucent plaques. This was significantly greater than the 2.4% rate for patients with echogenic plaque.

Histologic evaluation of heterogeneous carotid artery plaques reveals various amounts of IPH, lipids, cholesterol crystals, and loose stroma.[10] Some investigators have identified an amorphous lipid substance instead of hemorrhage in heterogeneous plaques. Lipids and hemorrhage appear similar by ultrasound, and it is not possible with our present technology to accomplish in vivo identification of these sonolucent areas. It has been reported that increased lipid concentration in and of itself makes a carotid artery plaque unstable.[11] Because both lipids and hemorrhage have been associated with symptoms, echolucency seems to indicate that the carotid plaque has a tendency to produce symptoms, regardless of its composition.

ULCERATION OF CAROTID PLAQUE

The blood-plaque interface has been characterized as smooth or ulcerated. Irregularity of the surface has been described on inspection of the plaque, either at the time of endarterectomy or on histologic sectioning. Moore and co-workers proposed a classification system based on the area of an ulcer, based on angiographic identification.[12, 13] Ulcers were designated as group A if less than 10 mm², group B if between 10 and 40 mm², or group C

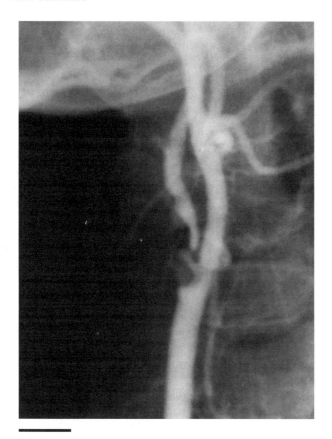

FIGURE 1.
Angiographic evidence of deep ulceration in a carotid artery plaque.

if larger than 40 mm^2. Figure 1 demonstrates an ulcer that would typically be characterized as group C.

Imparato and co-workers[4] could demonstrate no significance between symptomatic patients with ulcerated plaques identified by angiography compared with asymptomatic patients who also had ulcers. They found no correlation between degree of stenosis and ulcer occurrence.

In a study of 659 symptomatic patients from NASCET, Eliasziw and associates[14] found arteriographic evidence of ulceration in 230 plaques. In the group of patients treated medically, those with ulceration and a higher degree of stenosis had an increased risk of stroke.

O'Donnell et al.[15] compared specimens from 89 CEAs with preoperative arteriography and ultrasound. Using the definition of an

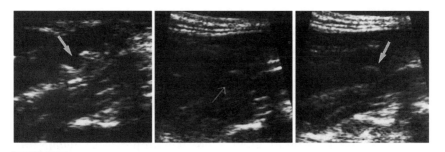

FIGURE 2.
Duplex ultrasound of a heterogeneous plaque with an ulcerated appearance in the **left panel,** either an ulcer or an echolucent area with a thin echogenic cap in the **middle panel,** and a juxtaluminal echolucent area consistent with intraplaque hemorrhage in the **right panel.**

ulcerated plaque as one with an irregular surface with punched out characteristics, they found a greater sensitivity of ultrasound (89%) than with angiography (59%), with similar specificities.

O'Leary and his group[16] were not able to confirm the sensitivity of ultrasound to predict ulceration on endarterectomy specimens, finding only 39% sensitivity.

Their definition of an ulcer was a surface irregularity of 1 mm^2 on macroscopic examination.

A number of factors may contribute to the disparity found in the literature with regard to the accuracy of identification and the significance of plaque ulceration. One is the variety of definitions used by authors, making it difficult to compare their results. A second factor is the degree of carotid stenosis, which some have reported as related to the presence of ulceration, or related to the ability to detect an ulcer with duplex ultrasound. A third factor is the timing of the investigation with regard to symptoms, because it has been observed that surface characteristics of plaque may change with time, and small ulcerated areas may later become smooth.

The sensitivity of ultrasound to identify ulcers may vary from 30% to 90%, in a review of the literature by Merritt and Bluth.[3] These authors have also observed that the majority of patients with ulcers identified by ultrasound have heterogeneous plaques, and that plaques with a homogeneous appearance usually have no ulcers. Ulceration and IPH seem to coexist in echolucent, heterogeneous plaques. It may be difficult to distinguish between IPH with a thin fibrous cap and ulceration, which in fact may be part of a continuum of plaque breakdown. Figure 2 shows three examples taken during one ultrasound study of the same patient in which the same plaque appears as an ulcer and as a hetereogenous IPH. These kinds of observations have led Lusby[5] to conclude that duplex scanning can detect degree of stenosis and morphologic appearance as relates to echogenicity, but may as yet be unable to accurately identify ulceration.

It appears that plaque heterogeneity indicates a certain degree of internal instability. The natural history and pathophysiology of plaque heterogeneity remains to be elucidated. It is not known whether progression of atherosclerosis within carotid plaque proceeds, as in other areas of the vascular tree, with an increase in the echolucent area, reflecting necrosis of plaque components or hemorrhage from within the wall or from the lumen. It would appear that heterogeneous plaques should be followed more closely than homogeneous ones, and that whatever the mechanism, a sudden increase in echolucency should be of concern.

CASE 1

Man, 70, with a history of diabetes and remote myocardial infarction was neurologically asymptomatic. He was followed with duplex ultrasonography for bilateral heterogeneous carotid artery plaques that remained stable at less than 50% stenosis. He had a TIA with right upper extremity weakness, which completely resolved. A new ultrasound was performed that demonstrated a change in the left carotid artery, with an increase of the degree of stenosis to at least 50% and probably closer to 70%. The character of the plaque was also noted to change, with the appearance of a large, echolucent area close to the lumen. A magnetic resonance angiogram (MRA) was obtained before surgery, which identified a stenosis of greater than 70%, with the appearance of IPH (Fig 3). Because of the character of the plaque on both the ultrasound and the MRA, surgery was performed the following day. Inspection of the plaque at the time of surgery confirmed the presence of a large area of IPH. Histologic examination of the plaque also noted the presence of areas of mural thrombus in addition to the large area of IPH.

COMMENT

It has been reported that acute hemorrhage is more often associated with neurologic symptoms than older hemorrhage on histologic examination of carotid artery specimens.[5] Although recent hemorrhage inside a plaque might progress to carotid occlusion and possible hemodynamic stroke, it more likely contributes to plaque instability at the luminal surface with subsequent cerebral embolization. In this patient, the appearance of symptoms seemed to correlate with the change in plaque morphology. It is reasonable

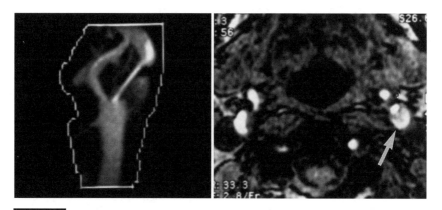

FIGURE 3.

Magnetic resonance angiogram showing a narrowed carotid artery lumen with evidence of intraplaque hemorrhage. The source image on the **right** demonstrates the narrow lumen seen on the **left,** as well as bright signals in the wall of the artery *(arrow)* that correspond to intramural hemorrhage.

to follow up more closely those patients with heterogeneous plaques until we better understand those specific characteristics that contribute to embolic activity. It is also reasonable to perform CEA expeditiously on those patients whose symptoms correlate with changes in the plaque.

Intraplaque hemorrhage is not usually as readily evident with MRA studies as with ultrasound because current MR technology does not allow in vivo identification of heterogeneous plaque to an acceptable degree of accuracy. The blood seen within the wall on the MRA source images in Figure 3 resembles that seen in a dissection within the wall of the artery. Whether this type of clear demonstration of IPH on MRA is associated with a greater degree of plaque instability is not known.

Another area for future investigation involves the role of antiplatelet or anticoagulant therapy in IPH. It is unclear whether such therapies stabilize the plaque or expand its hemorrhagic component, rendering it more susceptible to embolization.

In addition to the recognized neurologic end points of TIA and cerebral infarction, there are other indicators of plaque instability that are less overt. Evidence of retinal emboli by funduscopic examination and/or documentation of microemboli in the middle cerebral artery downstream from carotid artery pathology most probably represents emboli from an active and potentially symptomatic plaque at the carotid bifurcation. Further studies are needed to elucidate the natural history of such findings. Until such time as we have a better understanding of their clinical implications, the identification of asymptomatic embolic activity in association with heterogeneous plaque morphology warrants further attention.

The large randomized studies that have established degree of stenosis as the criterion upon which to recommend CEA have not focused on plaque morphology, and many questions remain regarding the best use of current information in treating our patients.

EMBOLI TO THE RETINA

Amaurosis fugax or transient monocular blindness is characterized as a sudden, brief episode of partial or complete dimming or obscuration of vision, lasting minutes to hours and followed by complete recovery. It is commonly caused by emboli that arise proximally in the cardiovascular system and travel to the retinal vessels. When significant and lasting hypoperfusion of retinal vasculature occurs, it causes a condition known as ocular ischemic syndrome. This may result from a large embolic load to the central retinal artery or from hypoperfusion associated with significant carotid artery stenosis or occlusion. While it is not possible to know the exact nature of emboli that travel to the brain, direct visualization of retinal emboli is possible by funduscopic examination.

Three types of retinal emboli have been observed in patients with transient or permanent retinal ischemia: cholesterol emboli, calcific emboli, and platelet-fibrin emboli. Cholesterol emboli are white, refractile lesions, usually seen at the bifurcation of an artery or arteriole. They may lodge for a period or pass across the retina quickly. These emboli originate from atherosclerotic plaques and have been designated Hollenhorst plaques. Calcific emboli, which originate from calcific cardiac valves, are seen as large white masses that lodge near the optic disc. Platelet-fibrin emboli, which are very difficult to see or photograph, also originate from atherosclerotic plaque. They appear as pale grayish particles, moving quickly through the arterial tree and causing evanescent visual symptoms.

Cholesterol emboli are not observed to occlude retinal vessels unless associated with platelet-fibrin embolic material. They are observed in patients who are both symptomatic and asymptomatic and are associated with an increased risk for stroke and vascular death.[17]

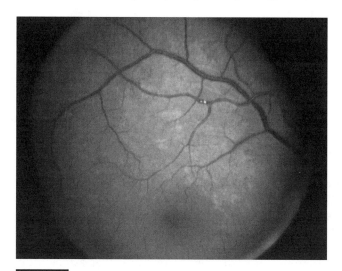

FIGURE 4.
Two cholesterol Hollenhorst plaques in a retinal branch artery.

Carotid stenosis is well recognized as a cause of retinal ischemia and visual symptoms, and recent investigators have turned their attention to the significance of associated plaque morphology. In a study designed to evaluate the relationship of retinal ischemia to plaque morphology, 165 patients who had symptoms of retinal ischemia were observed for 2–7 years (mean 3.3 years) with ultrasonographic evaluation of their extracranial carotid artery system.[18] Twenty-six percent of those studied had cerebrovascular or cardiovascular events in the follow-up period.

A significant association between complex heterogeneous plaque and subsequent vascular events was established, regardless of degree of carotid stenosis. The number of patients receiving antiplatelet therapy was similar in both groups, and a similar number of patients from each group underwent CEA based on severity of stenosis. These authors suggest that consideration be given to the morphologic appearance of the carotid plaque as well as to the degree of stenosis.

CASE 2
Man, 68, had a routine ophthalmologic examination. Two Hollenhorst plaques were observed in a branch artery of the right eye (Fig 4), while none were seen in the left eye. The patient had no symptoms of amaurosis fugax, but a faint bruit was auscultated at

the right carotid bifurcation. A duplex ultrasound was performed the next day, revealing a 50% to 70% stenosis on the right. The right carotid plaque was characterized as heterogeneous, with an irregular, ulcerated surface. The left ICA was less than 30% stenosed by ultrasound, and the plaque was primarily homogeneous.

The patient was active without cardiac symptoms. He reported no symptoms of TIA or stroke, and his cardiologic and neurologic examinations were normal. An MRA confirmed the degree of stenosis and did not detect any evidence of cerebral infarction. He underwent a right CEA at which time ulceration and IPH were seen. Histologic examination of the endarterectomy specimen demonstrated cholesterol clefts, calcification, and subintimal hemorrhage. In one area of the atheromatous intima, there was evidence of old, organized intimal hemorrhage or possibly mural thrombus, and adherent to this area was a recent clot with fibrin and platelets.

COMMENT

Although the Asymptomatic Carotid Atherosclerosis Study indicates that patients without neurologic symptoms but with carotid artery stenoses greater than 60% benefit from CEA, it is the author's practice to perform surgery primarily in those patients who have a more severe stenosis, closer to 80% or 90% and minimal cardiac risk factors. A subset of asymptomatic patients, as represented by this case, have heterogeneous plaque and retinal emboli, suggesting an active plaque with the potential for further downstream embolization. For patients in this subgroup whose surgical risk profile is good, particularly from a cardiac standpoint, the author would consider CEA for stenoses greater than 50%, because the ultrasound category is frequently designated as 50% to 70% stenosis, and it is not always possible to differentiate exactly 60%. For patients whose surgical risk profile is poorer and for those with stenoses of less than 50%, the author would observe the degree of stenosis, plaque morphology, and funduscopic examination for further changes with the patient on antiplatelet therapy.

For those patients with calcific or bilateral retinal emboli, investigation of more proximal cardiac or great vessel sources would be recommended.

It is well documented that the risk of stroke in patients with transient monocular blindness is less than in patients with other forms of TIA. These patients also have a greater risk of dying of myocardial infarction than of stroke. Although there is not a great deal of data about patients with asymptomatic retinal emboli, it may be safe to assume that they are at a somewhat increased risk of stroke, although consideration must be given to their cardiac risk. Patients in this category must therefore be carefully selected for CEA.

TRANSCRANIAL DOPPLER

Transcranial Doppler ultrasound (TCD) has been used throughout the world since 1982 to insonate intracranial vessels. This technology not only permits measurement of flow velocity in the intracranial arteries, but also has the capability to detect microembolic signals. Figure 5 is taken from the screen of a TCD monitor and demonstrates a typical embolus.

Studies have shown that these microembolic signals are composed of platelets, fibrinogen, cholesterol, and gaseous material. They have been observed in the ipsilateral middle cerebral artery

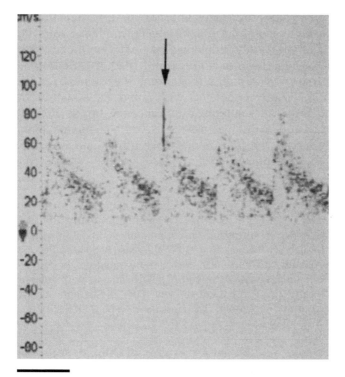

FIGURE 5.

A typical microembolus *(arrow)* appearing within the flow velocity waveform as detected by transcranial Doppler.

of patients with carotid stenosis, as well as during surgical procedures such as CEA and coronary artery bypass.[19]

In a study of patients with asymptomatic severe ICA stenosis who were prospectively followed up, Siebler and co-workers[20] found a significant association between a microembolic count of greater than 2 per hour and the occurrence of subsequent cerebral or retinal ischemic events. Our group has shown that microembolic signals were more common within the territories of symptomatic arteries, particularly those with severely stenotic lesions. In a follow-up study, recurrent ischemic events were more common within the distribution of arteries with TCD-detected microembolism and previous symptoms of cerebral or retinal ischemia.[21]

Other investigators have found similar correlation between plaque morphology and microembolic signals as detected by TCD. Valton et al.[22] showed that microembolic signals were significantly associated with plaque ulceration and not degree of stenosis, using the angiographic criteria of NASCET. Examination of the endarterectomy plaque by Sitzer and co-workers[23] led this group to conclude that ulceration and luminal thrombosis were the main source of cerebral emboli detected by TCD. Gaunt and associates[24] investigated whether unstable carotid plaques, so designated by preoperative color duplex ultrasound and postoperative histologic examination, were associated with microembolization by TCD. They concluded that embolization detected during the initial dissection phase of CEA was associated with ulcerated plaque and mural thrombus, but that preoperative ultrasound was not able to identify these characteristics.

> CASE 3
> Man, 64, with diabetes, had undergone a right CEA 2 years ago and was taking 325 mg of aspirin (1 aspirin tablet) daily. Routine surveillance duplex ultrasound revealed a normal postoperative right carotid artery with less than 30% stenosis. A 50% to 70% stenosis, probably closer to 50%, was demonstrated on the left, resulting from a plaque characterized as heterogeneous with a deeply ulcerated surface. The patient did not have any cerebral or cardiac symptoms and was otherwise considered to be a good surgical candidate.

The patient underwent a transcranial Doppler study in which both middle cerebral arteries were insonated for 30 minutes. Significant microembolic activity was noted on the left; no microemboli were found on the right side. The patient underwent a left CEA with intraoperative electroencephalographic and TCD monitoring. During dissection of the carotid artery before clamping, microemboli were detected. Surgical technique was altered based on this information and the microembolic signals abated. Upon inspection of the plaque when the artery was opened, an ulcerated surface with mural thrombus within the ulcer was noted. After completion of the procedure, the patient was again monitored in the recovery room and no further microemboli were detected. Pathologic examination of the specimen detected both intramural and luminal evidence of hemorrhage.

COMMENT

The presence of microembolic signals detected by TCD monitoring ipsilateral to an ulcerated, heterogeneous plaque indicates a degree of plaque activity and instability. While natural history studies would suggest that a heterogeneous plaque would be more likely to become symptomatic than an echogenic plaque, when coupled with microembolic activity as detected by TCD, consideration for surgery in a patient with a good surgical risk profile is more compelling.

Intraoperative TCD monitoring can provide the surgeon with information about microembolic activity.[19] A number of investigators have reported on the significance of perioperative microemboli as well as improved outcome when these microemboli were minimized. It is presumed that the microemboli detected in the middle cerebral artery during dissection originated from the mural thrombus subsequently noted on inspection of the plaque.

CONCLUSION

Duplex ultrasonography is now the most widely used imaging modality for the evaluation of carotid artery plaques because it provides information not only about the degree of stenosis, but also about plaque morphology. Current studies indicate that echolucent, heterogeneous carotid artery plaques are associated with neurologic symptoms, presumably caused by increased embolic activity from the plaque. Patients with these heterogeneous plaques who also demonstrate embolic activity by either funduscopic examination of the retinal arteries or TCD examination of the middle cerebral artery represent a group intermediate between symptomatic and asymptomatic patients. Recognizing that they may be at higher risk for neurologic symptoms, they should be considered for surgery, depending on assessment of their surgical risk. Additional long-term studies and further technological development are needed to determine which morphologic characteristics are associated with stroke risk and under what circumstances surgical intervention would be most beneficial.

REFERENCES

1. North American Symptomatic Carotid Endarterectomy Trial Collaborators: Beneficial effect of carotid endarterectomy in symptomatic patients with high-grade carotid stenosis. *N Engl J Med* 325:445–453, 1991.
2. Executive Committee for the Asymptomatic Carotid Atherosclerosis Study: Endarterectomy for asymptomatic carotid artery stenosis. *JAMA* 273:445–453, 1995.
3. Merritt C, Bluth E: Ultrasound identification of plaque composition, in Labs K (ed): *Diagnostic Vascular Ultrasound.* London, Edward Arnold, 1992, pp 213–224.
4. Imparato AM, Riles TS, Mintzer R, et al: The importance of hemorrhage in the relationship between gross morphologic characteristics and cerebral symptoms in 376 carotid artery plaques. *Ann Surg* 197:195–203, 1983.
5. Lusby RJ: Plaque characterization: Does it identify high risk groups?, in Bernstein EF, Callow AD, Nicolaides AN, et al (eds): *Cerebral Vascularization.* London, Med-Orion, 1993, pp 93–107.
6. Gray-Weale AC, Graham JC, Burrett JR, et al: Carotid artery atheroma: Comparison of preoperative B-mode ultrasound appearance with carotid endarterectomy specimen pathology. *J Cardiovasc Surg* 29:676–681, 1988.
7. Sterpetti AV, Schultz RD, Feldhaus RJ, et al: Ultrasonographic features of carotid plaque and the risk of subsequent neurologic defects. *Surgery* 104:652–660, 1988.
8. Geroulakos G, Domjan J, Nicolaides A, et al: Ultrasonic carotid artery plaque structure and the risk of cerebral infarction on computed tomography. *J Vasc Surg* 20:263–266, 1994.
9. Bock RW, Gray-Weal AC, Mock PA, et al: The natural history of asymptomatic carotid artery disease. *J Vasc Surg* 17:160–169, 1993.
10. Reilly LM, Lusby RJ, Hughes L, et al: Carotid plaque morphology using real time ultrasonography. Clinical and therapeutic implications. *Am J Surg* 146:188–193, 1983.
11. Feeley TM, Leen EJ, Colgan MP, et al: Histologic characteristics of carotid artery plaque. *J Vasc Surg* 13:719–724, 1991.
12. Moore WS, Boren C, Malone JM, et al: Natural history of nonstenotic asymptomatic ulcerative lesions of the carotid artery. *Arch Surg* 113:1352–1359, 1978.
13. Dixon S, Pais SO, Raviola C, et al: Natural history of nonstenotic, asymptomatic ulcerative lesions of the carotid artery. A further analysis. *Arch Surg* 117:1493–1497, 1982.

14. Eliasziw M, Streifler JV, Fox JA: Significance of plaque ulceration in symptomatic patients with high grade carotid stenosis. *Stroke* 25:305–308, 1994.

15. O'Donnell TF, Erodes L, Mackey WC, et al: Correlation of B-mode ultrasound imaging and arteriography with pathologic findings at carotid endarterectomy. *Arch Surg* 120:443–449, 1985.

16. O'Leary DH, Holen J, Ricotta JJ, et al: Carotid bifurcation disease: Prediction of ulceration with B-mode US. *Radiology* 162:523–525, 1987.

17. Bruno A, Russell PW, Jones WL, et al: Concomitants of asymptomatic retinal cholesterol emboli. *Stroke* 23:900–902, 1992.

18. O'Farrell CM, FitzGerald DE: Prognostic value of carotid ultrasound lesion morphology in retinal ischaemia: Result of a long term follow up. *Br J Ophthalmol* 77:781–784, 1993.

19. Babikian VL, Cantelmo NL: Clinical application of microemboli detection in cerebrovascular disease, in Klinghofer JK, Bartels E, Ringelstein EB (eds): *New Trends in Cerebral Hemodynamics and Neurosonology.* Amsterdam, Elsevier, 1997, pp 385–392.

20. Seibler M, Nachtman A, Sitzer M, et al: Cerebral microembolism and the risk of ischemia in asymptomatic high grade internal carotid artery stenosis. *Stroke* 26:2184–2186, 1995.

21. Babikian VL, Wijman CAC, Hyde C, et al: Cerebral microembolism and early recurrent cerebral or retinal ischemic events. *Stroke* 28:314–318, 1997.

22. Valton L, Larrue V, Arrue P, et al: Asymptomatic cerebral embolic signals in patients with carotid stenosis. Correlation with appearance of plaque ulceration on angiography. *Stroke* 26:813–815, 1995.

23. Sitzer M, Muller W, Seibler M, et al: Plaque ulceration and lumen thrombus are the main sources of cerebral microemboli in high-grade internal carotid artery stenosis. *Stroke* 26:1231–1233, 1995.

24. Gaunt ME, Brown L, Hartshorne T, et al: Unstable carotid plaques: Preoperative identification and association with intraoperative embolism detected by transcranial Doppler. *Eur J Vasc Endovasc Surg* 11:78–82, 1996.

PART II

Aortic Disease

CHAPTER 2

Management of Complications of Aortic Dissection

David C. Brewster, M.D.
Clinical Professor of Surgery, Massachusetts General Hospital and
Harvard Medical School, Boston, Massachusetts

Although significant advances in the diagnosis and treatment of acute aortic dissection have occurred during the last five decades, this condition remains a relatively frequent and highly morbid clinical event.[1] Indeed, acute aortic dissection is the most common lethal catastrophe involving the aorta, with an incidence surpassing that of ruptured abdominal aortic aneurysm (AAA).[2, 3] The misconception that ruptured AAA is more common results from the fact that most patients with AAA survive long enough to be seen by physicians, whereas those with acute dissection often die immediately or are misdiagnosed as having died of other causes of sudden death, such as acute myocardial infarction and cardiac arrhythmias.

The initiating mechanism in acute aortic dissection is a tear in the aortic intima through which blood surges into the media, separating aortic intima from adventitia. Dissections usually propagate from the intimal tear distally in the aorta, although retrograde extension can occur. The origin of any arterial trunk arising from the aorta may be compromised or the aortic valve rendered incompetent. Blood in the false channel can reenter the true aortic lumen anywhere along the course of the dissecting process, or external rupture may occur. Rupture of the aorta, the most common cause of death, occurs most frequently into the pericardial space or left pleural cavity. Timely diagnosis is important, because approximately 65% to 75% of patients with untreated acute aortic dissection die within the first 2 weeks after onset.[4, 5]

DIAGNOSIS

Although refinement in diagnostic modalities has clearly contributed to improved outcome during the past decade, an appropriate index of suspicion remains the key to rapid diagnosis. Severe chest or back pain leading to presentation for treatment within hours of onset is reported by more than 90% of patients.[1] Pulse deficits can be a helpful finding on physical examination. Because symptoms referable to aortic branch occlusion (e.g., abdominal pain from mesenteric ischemia or acute lower-extremity ischemia) may rapidly supersede back pain, the vascular surgeon may be the first to see the patient and have the opportunity to establish the diagnosis. We have found that about 10% of patients with dissections have primary complaints of lower extremity ischemia.[6]

Diagnostic confusion with acute coronary syndromes is usually eliminated with appropriate electrocardiography, and findings on plain chest radiography are generally not helpful. Although contrast arteriography was previously the diagnostic procedure of choice, graft replacement of the ascending aortic for acute dissection is frequently undertaken in contemporary practice without it. Rapid diagnosis in the emergency department can readily be made with transesophageal echocardiography (TEE), rapid-sequence dynamic CT, or MRI.[7] However, even after the diagnosis is confirmed by any of these imaging modalities, aortography is often desirable, particularly in dissections extending more distally, to (1) assess the degree of aortic insufficiency, if any; (2) assess the distal extent of dissection; (3) demonstrate the presence of aortic branch obstruction and compromise of blood flow to vital organs such as the bowel or kidneys; (4) clarify the mechanism of branch vessel occlusion and which dissection channel (true or false lumens) various aortic branches arise from; and (5) illustrate where points of spontaneous reentry may have already occurred between the two lumens. Such anatomical information is often invaluable in determining optimal forms of subsequent treatment.

INFLUENCE OF CLASSIFICATION ON MANAGEMENT

A key component in determining optimal therapy for patients with acute aortic dissection is the anatomical extent of the pathologic process. Patients with involvement of the ascending aorta or aortic arch in the dissection process, irrespective of the extent of involvement beyond the left subclavian artery, are considered to have *proximal* dissection (DeBakey classifications I and II, Stanford classification type A). Those patients with aortic dissection originating beyond the left subclavian artery and involving variable extents of the descending thoracic and/or abdominal aorta, and without involvement of the proximal aorta are classified as having *distal* dissection (DeBakey types III A and B, Stanford type B).

It is well established that the major risk of early death from acute aortic dissection relates to central complications, including acute rupture of the aorta into the mediastinum or pleural cavity, rupture into the pericardium causing acute tamponade, acute aortic valvular insufficiency with compromise of left ventricular function, or interference with coronary blood flow causing myocardial ischemia or infarction. Such potentially lethal events are much more common in dissections involving the proximal aorta and account for the current generally accepted approach of immediate direct surgical repair of the ascending aorta and/or aortic arch in patients with proximal dissections, even if more distal segments of the aorta are involved. Hence, since the initial introduction of surgical repair of aortic dissection by DeBakey and colleagues in 1955,[8] the evolution of thought and practice in the treatment of acute aortic dissection has gradually shifted toward definitive central repair of the aortic tear by cardiothoracic surgeons, with increasingly successful results.[5, 9–12]

In contrast, perhaps because of aortic structural differences as well as different dP/dt profiles, distal aortic dissections are considerably less likely to rupture in the acute phase. Hence, optimal therapy in patients with acute type B (DeBakey types III A and B) dissection remains much more controversial.[13–15] Indeed, in these forms of aortic dissection, vascular surgeons are most likely to become involved with patient management, clinical decision-making, and potential operative intervention.[16]

OPTIONS FOR TREATMENT OF DISTAL DISSECTIONS

While proximal aortic dissections are currently operated upon emergently by direct repair in most centers, a wider variety of approaches is possible for those patients with distal dissection. In some centers, early direct thoracic aortic repair of even uncomplicated distal dissections is felt to provide the best overall outcome.[12, 17] Graft replacement is performed via left thoracotomy from just distal to the left subclavian origin, presumably just proximal to the site of the initiating intimal tear, to the mid or distal thoracic aorta, including the tear and portion of the distal aorta dilated more than 4 cm in diameter. The aorta is transected circumferentially and the intimal septum sutured to the outer advential layers so that the true lumen is reperfused and false channel is obliterated. Use of Teflon felt pledgets or strips is often helpful to reapproximate the two lumens and to increase the strength and integrity of the suture line and anastomosis in those fragile tissues.

Although results of early graft repair of acute distal (type B) dissections have improved in the last decade, compared with earlier eras, operative mortality remains significant, ranging from 10% to 25%, depending upon the individual series reported.[11, 12, 17, 18] This frequently reflects the fact that dissection often occurs in older, severely hypertensive patients with multiple comorbid medical problems. Although highly dependent upon individual preferences, which vary considerably among centers, immediate direct repair for acute type B dissection is probably best limited to younger, good-risk patients in whom early surgical replacement of the diseased aortic segment theoretically may confer the best long-term protection by decreasing the incidence of subsequent aneurysmal dilation, extension of the dissection, or late ischemic complications.[13, 15] It is also generally agreed that acute distal dissections in patients with Marfan's syndrome should be treated surgically.[1]

In most centers, the consensus is that *initial medical management* of uncomplicated distal dissection is preferred and will provide a better outcome.[1, 11, 14] The rationale for medical management in patients with distal dissections is based on the following observations:

1. Proper drug therapy reduces the major forces tending to increase the dissection and its disastrous sequelae.
2. Medical therapy successfully prevents early death in the majority of patients.
3. Even contemporary operative mortality of immediate surgical therapy remains relatively high, because these patients are usually elderly with significant comorbid diseases.
4. The long-term outcome has been similar in surgically and medically treated patients with distal dissections.

Medical therapy is continued unless indications for surgery develop. As first described by Wheat and colleagues in 1965, the aim of early and long-term medical treatment is to control both the blood pressure and the force of ejection of blood from the heart by lowering dP/dt.[19] Both of these objectives help to prevent further extension of dissection, as well as progressive aortic dilatation and rupture. All patients should be managed initially in an ICU setting with full monitoring. Intravenous administration of a fast-acting agent (nitroprusside, arfonad) is required to reduce cardiac output and blood pressure to the lowest possible level consistent with maintaining cerebral, coronary, and renal perfusion. Simultaneously, to reduce dP/dt acutely, an intravenous β-blocker (propranolol, esmolol, metoprolol) is administered until there is evidence of satisfactory β-adrenergic blockade, as indicated by a pulse rate of less than 70 beats/min. Calcium channel antagonists (diltiazem, nifedipine) can be used if other measures fail, because these agents lower blood pressure and decrease dP/dt as well.

Although medical therapy generally suffices in the acute treatment of type B dissections, aortic rupture did occur in 10% of distal dissection cases in our review.[6] Therefore, an important component of initiating and following the progress of medical therapy is the size of the proximal descending thoracic aorta. In patients with significant (> 5 cm) aneurysmal dilation at the site of the aortic tear, consideration for early graft replacement is appropriate. In addition, when acute dissection occurs in continuity with a preexisting degenerative aortic aneurysm, the risk of rupture is high and graft replacement is the appropriate therapy.[20]

Once patients are stable and pain free with good blood pressure and pulse rate control, IV medications can be gradually withdrawn and oral antihypertensive and negative inotropic medications begun. Careful follow-up is mandatory, and serial chest x-rays and CT scans are required to monitor aortic size and detect progressive chronic aneurysmal formation of the false channel.

SELECTIVE SURGICAL THERAPY FOR COMPLICATIONS OF DISSECTION

If initial medical management of distal aortic dissections proves unsuccessful or complications of the dissection occur, selective surgical therapy by either direct graft repair of the aorta or peripheral surgical repair of obstructed aortic branches may be undertaken. With such a selective approach, surgical repair is reserved for patients who have (1) continuous pain; (2) evidence of bleeding; (3) progressive aneurysmal dilatation of the dissected aortic segment of more than 5 cm; or (4) evidence of peripheral vascular complications. The latter is a relatively frequent complication of aortic dissection, as the incidence of obstruction of major aortic branches causing malperfusion of the lower extremities, kidneys, or major abdominal visceral organs is approximately 33% in acute aortic dissections. Indeed, such aortic branch occlusion may some-

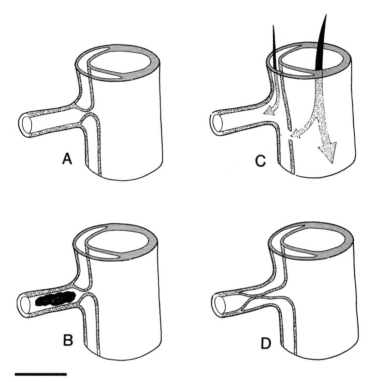

FIGURE 1.

Mechanism of aortic branch obstruction in acute dissection. Bulging of the false lumen can produce occlusion at the branch orifice **(A).** The subsequent thrombosis distally may occur **(B).** Intimal detachment at the branch orifice may occur with perfusion largely via the false channel **(C).** The dissection process may also proceed into the branch, causing obstruction beyond the actual branch orifice **(D).** (Courtesy of Cambria RP, Brewster DC, Gertler J, et al: Vascular complications associated with spontaneous aortic dissection. *J Vasc Surg* 7:199–209, 1988.)

times constitute the principal mode of presentation, or become the primary focus of treatment in some patients.[2, 6, 21, 22]

MECHANISM OF AORTIC BRANCH OBSTRUCTION

The most common mechanism of vessel obstruction involves extrinsic compression of the true arterial lumen by the bulging dissected false lumen, thereby compromising or obstructing flow to the vascular territory perfused by the branch vessel.[2, 6] This process may be circumferential at a branch vessel orifice or it may extend for varying distances into the particular branch (Fig 1). On other occasions, the ostium of a branch vessel may be obstructed

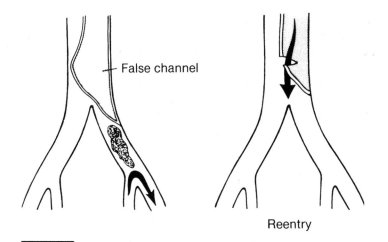

FIGURE 2.

Compromise of true lumen by dissection channel producing distal aortic obstruction. This may be complicated by distal thrombosis or relieved by spontaneous (or surgical) reentry. (Courtesy of Brewster DC, Cambria RP: Role of the vascular surgeon in the management of dissecting aortic aneurysms, in Veith FJ (ed): *Current Critical Problems in Vascular Surgery.* St Louis, Quality Medical Publishing, 1989, pp 291–302.)

by disrupted intimal flaps or intussusception of detached intima into the proximal aspect of the branch artery. Rarely, embolic occlusion of vessels remote from the dissection process may occur secondary to discharge of clot from the false lumen.[22] Such embolic material may originate at either the site of the initiating intimal tear or at a more distal point of reentry.

In addition to possible compromise of branch vessel origins by the dissection, if branch vessel flow obstruction is complete, in situ thrombosis formation distal to the point of occlusion may occur secondary to stasis. In these circumstances, branch obstruction may persist despite correction of the dissection by proximal thoracic aortic repair. Similarly, continued obstruction of branch orifices by persistent intimal flaps or remote embolization may persist despite redirection of flow into the true lumen by initial central repair. These circumstance explain why primary aortic repair may not always relieve the peripheral vascular complications of aortic dissection, and emphasize that additional methods of revascularization may occasionally be required for a successful outcome.

Spontaneous reentry of the false lumen (Fig 2) may relieve obstruction in the true lumen and account for the fluctuating clinical picture of visceral or peripheral ischemic manifestations often noted in patients with acute dissection.[1] Reentry commonly occurs at points where aortic tributaries are sheared off or may occur spontaneously at one or more points along the extent of the dissection. Reentry provides communication between the true and false lumens, and allows the potential for double-channel distal perfusion or continued adequate perfusion of certain aortic branches solely from the false lumen. Indeed, this concept provides the rationale for the surgical procedure of fenestration, to be discussed subsequently.

INCIDENCE OF VASCULAR COMPLICATIONS

Peripheral vascular complications of aortic dissection are relatively common, noted in from 20% to 50% of patients with acute aortic dissection in various series in the literature.[2, 6, 9, 21, 22] The frequency of branch vessel obstruction will vary, depending upon both the distribution and extent of dissection and the method of diagnosis. If one uses the classification of DeBakey et al.,[9] peripheral vascular complications are understandably more common with more extensive type I and III B dissections that involve areas of the aorta from which major visceral or extremity branches originate, as opposed to dissections confined to the ascending or descending thoracic aorta (DeBakey type II and III A) that potentially involve only intercostal and spinal arteries. Thus, in our report of the Massachusetts General Hospital experience,[6] peripheral vascular complications were noted in 33% of all 345 patients with aortic dissection, but occurred in approximately 50% of patients with type I and III B dissections, in contrast to only 10% with type II and III A lesions.

Similarly, evolution and changes in diagnostic methods used in evaluations of patients with suspected aortic dissection will influence the incidence of documented peripheral vascular complications. For example, the report of Hughes et al.[22] at Emory cited a 21% incidence of peripheral vascular complications in 86 cases of aortic dissection, substantially less than the approximately 30% incidence noted in several other large series focusing primarily on this topic.[6, _] As the Emory group acknowledges, however, angiography was used to diagnose or define the extent of dissection in only 22% of cases in their recent 5-year series. Transesophageal echocardiography (TEE), the most frequently (52%) used technique in their series, may be more expeditious and highly accurate in diagnosis of the condition, but does not examine the abdominal aorta or its branches. Likewise, MRI or CT scanning is not likely as sensitive for detection and demonstration of branch vessel involvement

TABLE 1.
Peripheral Vascular Complications of Aortic Dissection

Aortic or iliac artery obstruction with lower-extremity ischemia
Upper-extremity ischemia
Neurologic ischemic events
Mesenteric ischemia
Renal ischemia
Late aneurysm formation

as is angiography.[22] Hence, the incidence of peripheral vascular lesions may be underestimated with these diagnostic modalities.

CLINICAL MANIFESTATIONS OF VASCULAR COMPLICATIONS

Although the clinical picture of classic aortic dissection is well described and recognized, patients may vary considerably in their mode of presentation and clinical course. The variable origin and extent of the dissection process, with widely different resultant anatomical and physiologic ramifications, may cause a wide spectrum of clinical problems and sometimes diagnostic uncertainty. Indeed, the condition has often been referred to as "the great clinical masquerader."[2]

In most cases, a history of typical chest or back pain, longstanding hypertension, murmur of aortic insufficiency, widened mediastinum on chest x-ray, or symptoms referable to occlusion of aortic branch vessels will suggest the proper diagnosis. On occasion, however, an atypical presentation with primarily manifestations of a peripheral vascular complication may cause the vascular surgeon to be the first physician to evaluate the patient. For example, painless aortic dissection presenting with an acutely ischemic limb mimicking acute thromboembolic arterial occlusion is well recognized.[1, 6, 16, 23] The proper diagnosis may only be suspected after unsuccessful attempts to restore extremity circulation by catheter thromboembolectomy or findings of dissection at the arteriotomy site. Hence, it is important to make the correct diagnosis so that definitive diagnostic evaluation and therapy can be rapidly instituted.

A wide variety of both early and late vascular complications may affect the aorta or its major branches as a consequence of the initial aortic dissection (Table 1). Based upon a large autopsy series, iliac artery compromise is most common, followed in descending order by innominate, left common carotid, left subclavian, renal, superior mesenteric, and celiac involvement.[4] The sites of aortic branch occlusion and related clinical events in our series from the Massachusetts General Hospital of peripheral vascular complications associated with aortic dissection are shown in Figure 3.[6]

Lower-extremity Ischemia

The vascular surgeon is most likely to encounter a patient manifesting acute lower-extremity ischemic symptoms caused by compromise of flow in the abdominal aorta or iliac arteries (Fig 4). Because pulse deficits and distal perfusion are influenced by systemic blood pressure, the presence or absence of distal reentry, and possible oscillation of an intimal flap, typically physical findings and patient symptoms may wax and wane in the initial phases of acute dissection.[1] If the diagnosis of aortic dissection is not initially suspected and angiography is performed to evaluate acute lower extremity ischemia, it is important that characteristic arteriographic features of the process be recognized, thereby enabling a correct diagnosis to be established. As an aortic dissection progresses caudally from its thoracic origin, the false lumen tends to spiral around the long axis of the aorta, causing varying degrees of compression of the true lumen and resulting in a variable and often complex pattern of major aortic branches arising from either the true or false channels. Depending on placement of the arteriographic catheter tip and filming sequence, the narrowed true lumen may be the only vascular channel opacified, especially when dissection has extended to the iliofemoral region. Recognition may hinge on characteristic angiography findings, which, in addition to actual visualization of an intimal flap or double lumen, include several indirect signs suggestive of aortic dissection, such as (1) a relatively small opacified aortic lumen relative to that of the iliac arteries; (2) the absence of one or more lumbar vessels usually arising from the posterolateral abdominal aorta; or (3) the fusiform tapering of iliac or femoral arteries to a point of occlusion.[23] The last feature is particularly noteworthy because acute thrombotic or embolic occlusion usually results in abrupt vessel occlusion angiographically, whereas dissection typically produces a long, fusiform, tapered narrowing of the vessel proximal to the occlusion.

Upper-extremity Ischemia

Compromise of upper-extremity circulation secondary to innominate or subclavian artery obstruction by the dissection is also a relatively common observation. Indeed, asymmetry of upper extremity pulses and/or blood pressure is one of the classic physical findings suggesting the diagnosis of acute aortic dissection. As with

Distribution of Peripheral Vascular Complications

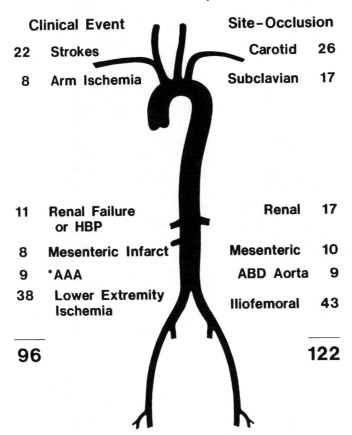

Clinical Event		Site-Occlusion	
22	Strokes	Carotid	26
8	Arm Ischemia	Subclavian	17
11	Renal Failure or HBP	Renal	17
8	Mesenteric Infarct	Mesenteric	10
9	*AAA	ABD Aorta	9
38	Lower Extremity Ischemia	Iliofemoral	43
96			**122**

*Aneurysm of abdominal or thoracoabdominal aorta resulting from dissection

FIGURE 3.

Sites and distribution of peripheral vascular complications and related clinical events of Massachusetts General Hospital study. Disparity between occlusions and clinical events reflects asymptomatic occlusions. (Courtesy of Cambria RP, Brewster DC, Gertler J, et al: Vascular complications associated with spontaneous aortic dissection. *J Vasc Surg* 7:199–209, 1988.)

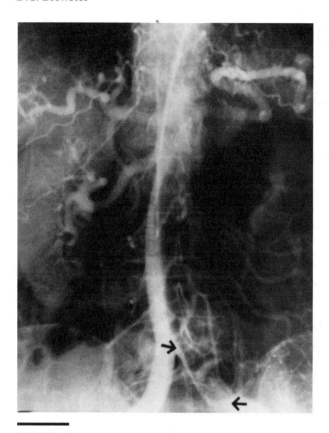

FIGURE 4.

Aortogram demonstrating marked narrowing of infrarenal aorta and near total occlusion of left common iliac artery *(arrows)* in patient with type I dissection. Ascending aortic repair restored left femoral pulse. (Courtesy of Brewster DC, Cambria RP: Role of the vascular surgeon in the management of dissecting aortic aneurysms, in Veith FJ (ed): *Current Critical Problems in Vascular Surgery.* St Louis, Quality Medical Publishing, 1989, pp 291–302.

other etiologies of upper-extremity arterial stenosis or occlusion, arm or hand ischemia is frequently not severe and often well tolerated because of availability of abundant collateral circulation.

Neurologic Events

Neurologic manifestations of aortic dissection most commonly represent transient ischemic attacks (TIAs), or stroke secondary to impairment of cerebral perfusion. While TIA or stroke may be related to discharge of thromboemboli from the proximal intimal tear, aortic arch, or at a reentry point in the carotid artery itself, most acute cerebrovascular events are attributable to obstruction of the true lumen of the innominate or carotid branches of the aortic arch by the dissection.

In addition to stroke or TIAs, lower-extremity neurologic manifestations may result from spinal cord injury or ischemic insult to peripheral nerves. Ischemic injury to the spinal cord, aside from its possible occurrence as a postoperative complication of direct surgical repair, may occur as a primary presenting event in a small percentage of patients with acute aortic dissection, and can be of diagnostic importance.[9]

Renal or Mesenteric Ischemia

Autopsy or arteriographic data reveal that approximately 10% of patients with acute aortic dissection will have impaired perfusion of major visceral or renal arteries.[4, 6, 9, 21] Clinically evident sequelae of such impaired perfusion are less common, however, with only 5% to 6% of patients demonstrating clinically significant intestinal or renal ischemia. This is fortunate, for both of these vascular complications of acute aortic dissection are highly significant determinants of poor outcome.[6, 12, 21] Despite successful definitive central aortic repair of the dissection, death often results from irreversible mesenteric infarction or acute renal failure.

Abdominal pain out of proportion to physical findings, as typically noted with acute mesenteric ischemia, should suggest probable involvement of the celiac and/or superior mesenteric artery in the acute aortic dissection and requires urgent attention. Renal artery involvement may be considerably more difficult to recognize. Several factors may cloud evaluation of potential renal artery compromise: (1) renal function abnormalities may be preexistent and unrelated to obstruction coincident with dissection; (2) a single renal artery occlusion may not be recognized, because adequate function is maintained by a normally perfused contralateral kidney; (3) renal arteries may be perfused form true or false lumens, or both, requiring contrast opacification of both channels to verify patency or obstruction; (4) renal artery obstruction may be incomplete, producing significant hypertension without infarction or ischemic nephropathy and renal failure; and (5) developing renal insufficiency or low urinary output may be more a consequence of systemic hypotension than mechanical interference with renal artery blood flow.

Oliguria, flank pain, or hematuria are of possible diagnostic importance, and should prompt immediate investigation. It must be emphasized that diagnostic modalities such as TEE or aortic CT and MRI studies may not elucidate the status of renal artery blood flow, and contrast arteriography may often be required in these circumstances. When renal artery compromise occurs in acute aortic dissection and is sufficient to cause acute functional deterioration, resultant mortality is quite high, similar to that with acute mesenteric ischemia.[6] Thus, urgent corrective measures are often required to preserve renal function and avoid a poor outcome.

Late Aneurysm Formation

Although acute aneurysmal change of the aorta and false lumen is rarely seen, subsequent frank aneurysmal dilation of the thoracoabdominal or infrarenal aorta to a degree requiring consideration for delayed surgical repair is not uncommon.[10, 11, 24] Indeed, 15% to 30% of late deaths occurring in patients with prior aortic dissection are caused by late rupture of the involved segment or another part of the aorta.[1] Such progressive aneurysmal dilation may occur in the aorta distal to even previously successful proximal graft repair of acute dissection, as many studies have indicated that the false lumen often remains patent via multiple points of distal reentry or by continued perfusion at the ostia or severed branches in a high percentage (approximately 85%) of patients.[25] Hence, careful lifelong follow-up by serial imaging studies of the aorta is imperative. In addition, careful medical supervision and blood pressure control is essential. For example, DeBakey et al. noted that later aneurysms of the thoracic, thoracoabdominal, or abdominal aorta developed in 45% of patients with poor blood pressure control, but in only 17% of those with well-controlled hypertension.[9] Similar findings have been emphasized by Neya et al.[26]

Thus, vascular surgeons may become involved with repair of such late aneurysmal dissections. Surgery is generally considered when symptoms occur or when progressive enlargement of the dissected aorta exceeds 6 cm in diameter.[2, 10] Chronic dissections constitute a reasonable proportion of patients in a series of thoracoabdominal aneurysm repair in many reports,[10, 11] and more localized repair of infrarenal aneurysms or even iliac aneurysms secondary to chronic dissections have been reported.[22, 23, 26, 27]

TREATMENT OF VASCULAR COMPLICATIONS

Several methods of revascularization are available to the vascular surgeon in the management of vascular complications of aortic dissection. A *fenestration procedure* has been well described in many reports and documented to effectively restore lower-extremity circulation, and lead to acceptable long-term survival when used as the only treatment modality.[6, 27-30] Similarly, by establishing effective communication between true and false lumens, it may also often successfully restore perfusion of compromised renal or visceral arteries and effectively treat acute mesenteric or renal ischemia. The principal appeal of fenestration is that it offers potential correction of life- or limb-threatening vascular complications of dissection by means of a procedure that likely causes less morbidity, because it does not entail thoracic aortic clamping, require any form of cardiopulmonary bypass, or expose the patient to the possibility of ischemic spinal cord injury.[28, 29]

The procedure is usually carried out in the infrarenal aorta, by a retroperitoneal approach if desired. The aorta is divided, and a portion of the proximal septum between the true and false lumens is excised, providing a reentry point and free communication of flow between the two channels (Fig 5). Most often, segmental graft insertion is carried out, although primary reanastomosis of the divided aorta may be done. Proximally, the suture line involves all three layers of the normal aortic wall in the portion of the aortic circumference uninvolved with dissection (true lumen) and only the aortic adventitia in that portion representing the false lumen. Use of pledgeted sutures may obviate many of the acknowledged problems of anastomosis involving such friable aortic tissue. Distally, the graft anastomosis may reapproximate both true and false lumens by incorporating both layers of the aortic wall in the distal suture line, or a distal anastomosis may be constructed at nondissected distal portions of the iliac or femoral vessels.

For lower-extremity ischemia involving only one extremity, caused by unilateral iliac obstruction, femorofemoral grafts offer an expedient and effective treatment, particularly in patients with otherwise uncomplicated distal (type III or B) dissections who may be treated preferentially by medical management.[6, 22] Use of axillobifemoral grafts has been described by Laas and colleagues[30] for patients with bilateral lower-extremity ischemia associated with compromise of the aortic lumen resulting from more chronic dissections. Extra-anatomical grafts may also be extremely useful in other locations as well; for example, correction of persistent upper-extremity ischemia after repair of proximal dissection by means of an axilloaxillary bypass. On occasion, carotid-carotid or subclavian-carotid bypass may be used for cerebral ischemia persisting after aortic repair, or if the existence of an acute neurologic deficit is felt to preclude immediate direct operation.[6]

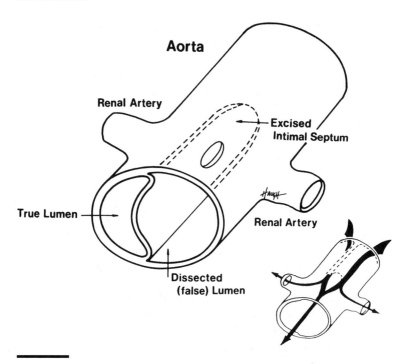

FIGURE 5.
Fenestration procedure. Aorta is divided distal to renal arteries, with true
and false lumens evident. Ellipse, or "window," of dissected intima is excised, and then graft is sutured end to end to composite lumen. (Courtesy
of Hunter JA, Dye WS, Javid H, et al: Abdominal aortic resection in thoracic dissection. *Arch Surg* 111:1258–1262. Copyright 1976, American
Medical Association.)

Relief of acute mesenteric or renal ischemia, either after initial
aorta repair that fails to adequately restore flow to these branches
or in selected patients as a primary intervention, may be accomplished by either a fenestration procedure or direct bypass grafting. Grafts to the visceral or renal vessels may originate from the
lower aspect of the infrarenal aorta if uninvolved with the dissection, or more commonly, from an uninvolved iliac artery. Alternatively, an aortic graft inserted as part of a fenestration procedure
may serve as an origin for such bypass grafts to renal or visceral
arteries if the surgeon does not feel confident enough that fenestration alone will adequately restore bowel or kidney perfusion. Renal artery reconstruction may also be readily achieved by hepato-
renal or splenorenal bypass grafts if the celiac origin is spared by

the dissection.[23] Use of renal autotransplantation has also been reported as a method of renal salvage in aortic dissection.

ENDOVASCULAR METHODS

The continued high morbidity and mortality of aortic dissection, particularly when associated with peripheral vascular complications, has spawned interest in development of alternative forms of therapy that may perhaps be less morbid and more expedient than conventional surgical approaches. This is particularly true of dissections complicated by ischemia of the kidneys and/or abdominal visceral, in which irreversible and often lethal renal or bowel infarction may occur within hours of onset.

In recent years, a number of reports have described percutaneous catheter-based endovascular approaches and their potential application and appeal in management of both acute and chronic dissections.[31–35] Balloon dilatation catheters may be used percutaneously to either enlarge small reentry points that are providing ineffective flow to end organs being exclusively perfused from the false channel, or, in some instances, actually establish *de novo* a point of reentry when these are absent, by fenestrating the septum between the true and false lumens, thereby providing satisfactory flow and alleviating ischemic manifestations. As with surgical fenestration, this approach can also be used to decompress the false lumen if it is encroaching significantly on the true aortic lumen, thereby improving antegrade flow to the lower extremities. Similarly, endovascular stents have been used to treat the site of initiating intimal tear itself, improve a compromised true aortic lumen, or improve flow in compromised major aortic branches.

Such techniques may be applied for vascular complications of subacute or chronic dissections, but perhaps have their greatest appeal as emergent therapies performed at the time of diagnostic angiography. In this fashion, they could potentially serve as valuable adjunctive measures by minimizing critical organ ischemic time, thereby improving the patient's prognosis for definitive thoracic aortic repair, or they could represent definitive therapy in some instances where nonoperative treatment of the dissection is judged preferable. Although current clinical experience is limited, such techniques appear to hold considerable promise as a potential treatment option in the management of certain complex high-risk patients.

CONCLUSION

Peripheral vascular complications occur in approximately one third of aortic dissections, as a consequence of compromise of major branch vessel flow by the dissection process. A variety of ischemic manifestations may occur, most often involving lower-extremity ischemia, but also potentially affecting the upper extremities, CNS, or circulation to the kidneys or intestines. Although direct thoracic repair of the dissection itself often corrects or alleviates the peripheral vascular complications, vascular surgical procedures may be necessary if branch vessel obstruction persists after thoracic aortic repair, or if the dissection is felt to be better treated by nonoperative management. In some patients, critical renal, mesenteric, or advanced lower-extremity ischemia may assume treatment priority. A variety of revascularization options are available. Newer endovascular treatment modalities appear to hold promise in the treatment of some of these complications.

REFERENCES

1. DeSanctis RW, Doroghazi RM, Austen WG, et al: Medical progress: Aortic dissection. *N Engl J Med* 317:1060–1067, 1987.
2. Walker PJ, Sarris GE, Miller DC: Peripheral vascular manifestations of acute aortic dissection, in Rutherford RB (ed): *Vascular Surgery.* Philadelphia, WB Saunders, 1995, pp 1087–1102.
3. Wheat MW Jr, Palmer RF: Dissecting aneurysms of the aorta. *Curr Probl Surg* July 1–43, 1971.
4. Hirst AE Jr, Johns VJ Jr, Kime SW Jr: Dissecting aneurysm of the aorta: A review of 505 cases. *Medicine* 37:217–279, 1958.
5. Miller DC: Surgical management of aortic dissections: Indications, perioperative management, and long-term results, in Doroghazi RM, Slater EE (eds): *Aortic Dissection.* New York: McGraw-Hill, 1983, pp 193–243.
6. Cambria RP, Brewster DC, Gertler J, et al: Vascular complications associated with spontaneous aortic dissection. *J Vasc Surg* 7:199–209, 1988.
7. Nienaber CA, Kodolitsch YV, Nicholas V, et al: The diagnosis of thoracic aortic dissection by noninvasive imaging procedures. *N Engl J Med* 328:1–9, 1993.
8. DeBakey ME, Cooley DA, Creech O Jr: Surgical considerations of dissecting aneurysms of the aorta. *Ann Surg* 142:586–612, 1955.
9. DeBakey ME, McCollum CH, Crawford ES, et al: Dissection and dissecting aneurysms of the aorta: Twenty-year follow-up of five hundred twenty-seven patients treated surgically. *Surgery* 92:1118–1134, 1982.
10. Crawford ES, Svensson LG, Coselli JS, et al: Aortic dissection and dissecting aortic aneurysms. *Ann Surg* 208:254–273, 1988.

11. Svensson LG, Crawford ES, Hess KR, et al: Dissection of the aorta and dissecting aortic aneurysms. *Circulation* 82:IV-24S–IV-38S, 1990.

12. Miller DC, Mitchell RS, Oyer PE, et al: Independent determinants of operative mortality for patients with aortic dissections. *Circulation* 70:I-153S–I-164S, 1984.

13. Miller DC: The continuing dilemma concerning medical versus surgical management of patients with acute type B dissections. *Semin Thorac Cardiovasc Surg* 5:33–46, 1993.

14. Glower DD, Famn JI, Speier RH, et al: Comparison of medical and surgical therapy for uncomplicated descending aortic dissection. *Circulation* 82:IV-39S–IV-46S, 1990.

15. Roberts CS, Roberts WC: Aortic dissection with the entrance tear in the descending thoracic aorta. *Ann Surg* 213:356–368, 1991.

16. Brewster DC: Role of the vascular surgeon in the management of dissecting aortic aneurysms, in Veith FJ (ed): *Current Critical Problems in Vascular Surgery*. St. Louis, Quality Medical Publishing, 1989, pp 291–302.

17. Fann JI, Smith JA, Miller DC, et al: Surgical management of aortic dissection during a 30-year period. *Circulation* 92:II-113S–II-121S, 1995.

18. Jex RK, Schaff HV, Piehler JM, et al: Early and late results following repair of dissections of the descending thoracic aorta. *J Vasc Surg* 3:226–237, 1986.

19. Wheat MW, Palmer RF, Bartley TB, et al: Treatment of dissecting aneurysms of the aorta without surgery. *J Thorac Cardiovasc Surg* 50:364–373, 1965.

20. Cambria RP, Brewster DC, Moncure AC, et al: Spontaneous aortic dissection in the presence of coexistent or previously repaired atherosclerotic aortic aneurysm. *Ann Surg* 208:619–624, 1988.

21. Fann JI, Sarris GE, Mitchell RS, et al: Treatment of patients with aortic dissection presenting with peripheral vascular complications. *Ann Surg* 212:705–713, 1990.

22. Hughes JD, Bacha EA, Dodson RF, et al: Peripheral vascular complications of aortic dissection. *Am J Surg* 170:209–212, 1995.

23. Brewster DC: Management of peripheral artery complications in patients with aortic dissection, in Yao JST, Pearce WH (eds): *Arterial Surgery: Management of Challenging Problems*. Stamford, Conn, Appleton and Lange, 1996, pp 247–264.

24. Glower DD, Speier RH, White WD, et al: Management and long-term outcome of aortic dissection. *Ann Surg* 214:31–41, 1991.

25. da Gama AD: The surgical management of aortic dissection: From uniformity to diversity, a continuous challenge. *J Cardiovasc Surg* 32:141–153, 1991.

26. Neya K, Omoto R, Kyo S, et al: Outcome of Stanford type B acute aortic dissection. *Circulation* 86:II-1S–II-7S, 1992.

27. Hunter JA, Dye WS, Javid H, et al: Abdominal aortic resection in thoracic dissection. *Arch Surg* 111:1258–1262, 1976.

28. Elefteriades JA, Hartleroad J, Gusberg RJ, et al: Long-term experience with descending aortic dissection: The complication-specific approach. *Ann Thorac Surg* 53:11–21, 1992.

29. Elefteriades JA, Hammond GL, Gusberg RJ, et al: Fenestration revisited: A safe and effective procedure for descending aortic dissection. *Arch Surg* 125:786–790, 1990.

30. Laas J, Heinemann M, Schaefers H-J, et al: Management of thoracoabdominal malperfusion in aortic dissection. *Circulation* 84:III-20S–III-24S, 1991.

31. Williams DM, Brothers TE, Messina LM: Relief of mesenteric ischemia in type III aortic dissection with percutaneous fenestration of the aortic septum. *Radiology* 174:450–452, 1990.

32. Walker PJ, Dake MD, Mitchell RS, et al: The use of endovascular techniques for the treatment of complications of aortic dissection. *J Vasc Surg* 18:1042–1051, 1993.

33. Slonim SM, Dake MD, Semba CP, et al: Aortic dissection: Percutaneous management of ischemic complications with endovascular stents and a balloon fenestration. *J Vasc Surg* 23:241–253, 1996.

34. Slonim SM, Miller DC, Dake MD: Endovascular techniques of treatment of complications of aortic dissection, in Yao JST, Pearce WH (eds): *Arterial Surgery: Management of Challenging Problems.* Stamford, Conn, Appleton and Lange, 1996, pp 283–289.

35. Slonim SM, Nyman UR, Semba CP, et al: True lumen obliteration in complicated aortic dissection: Endovascular treatment. *Radiology* 201:161–166, 1996.

CHAPTER 3

Treatment of Infected Aortic Grafts With In Situ Aortic Reconstruction Using Superficial Femoral-Popliteal Veins

Ryan T. Hagino, M.D.
Assistant Professor of Surgery, University of Texas Health Science Center at San Antonio; Attending Staff, Wilford Hall Medical Center, Lackland AFB, Texas

G. Patrick Clagett, M.D.
Pickens Professor of Medical Science, Chief of the Division of Vascular Surgery, University of Texas Southwestern Medical Center, Dallas, Texas

Since 1989, we have used autologous superficial femoral-popliteal vein (SFPV) as conduit for in situ aortoiliac reconstruction after excision of infected aortic prosthetic grafts.[1] However, use of the SFPV for vascular reconstruction is not a new concept. Initial experience with these veins was limited to major reconstructions of the superior vena cava; even when applied to the low-pressure, low-flow venous system, patency results for venous bypasses were exceptional.[2] Despite these initial successes in the 1950s, use of the SFPV as a bypass conduit has never become popular. This reluctance is probably based upon fears of excessive venous morbidity in the donor limb and difficulty in harvesting the autograft. In addition, SFPV grafts may become aneurysmal over time when placed in the high-pressure, high-flow aortoiliac system. Despite these concerns, we now routinely use SFPV autografts for in situ aortic reconstruction after excision of infected aortic grafts. This policy was adopted in an effort to overcome the problems associated with the traditional surgical management of infected aortic grafts, particularly secondary graft infection of extra anatomic bypasses, thrombosis of extra anatomic bypasses, and aortic stump dehiscence.

PREOPERATIVE PREPARATION

Preoperative work-up of patients with aortic graft infection is neither leisurely nor superficial. Diagnostic testing must be directed at localizing the site of infection, defining the anatomy of previous arterial reconstructions, and identifying critical vascular beds that will require revascularization after removal of the infected graft. A complete history and physical examination is mandatory and will provide invaluable information. For instance, a history of gastrointestinal bleeding may suggest graft-enteric communication, whereas bleeding from sinus tracts in the groin may indicate the presence of a contained ruptured anastomotic femoral false aneurysm. Of course, many patients' only complaint may be anorexia, weight loss, and lethargy. In addition to an accurate clinical history, a detailed surgical history must be obtained from the patient, previous medical records, and old operative reports. We have found it is common for a patient to have had many antecedent vascular procedures to treat prior graft failure or "localized" graft infection.[1, 3] Careful physical examination may reveal important findings that may influence operative management. For example, a pulsatile mass in the epigastrium may suggest a proximal anastomotic aortic pseudoaneurysm, whereas a pulsatile groin mass implies distal anastomotic dehiscence. Skin petechiae isolated to one limb may be a manifestation of septic emboli from a single limb of an infected bifurcated graft. A single draining sinus in an old groin incision may be the only manifestation of an indolent graft infection. Laboratory examination should include electrolytes, renal function tests, liver function tests, coagulation studies, urinalysis, blood cultures, and appropriately obtained wound cultures. Broad-spectrum antibiotics are initiated until antibiotic sensitivities of isolated organisms can be determined.

Initial diagnostic tests are usually directed at imaging the infected prosthesis in relationship to surrounding structures. We have used both contrast-enhanced CT and MRI. False aneurysms can be identified both at the proximal and distal anastomoses with these imaging techniques. Perigraft fluid collections may also be seen; extent of involvement may be seen isolated to an infected groin or involving the entire graft. On occasion, a psoas abscess or diverticular abscess may also be identified. Angiography is considered essential before intervention. As mentioned earlier, these patients have often had multiple prior vascular procedures both above and below the inguinal ligament. These prior procedures may complicate operative planning. Also, the extent of visceral, renal, pelvic, and infrainguinal vascular occlusive disease observed on angiogram may significantly influence the type of revascularization performed after graft excision; findings of significant occlusive disease in other regions will determine the need for concomitant visceral, renal, or infrainguinal reconstruction.

A vital part of preoperative testing before in situ autologous aortic reconstruction is extensive lower extremity venous duplex imaging. Duplex vein mapping allows preoperative determination of diameter and length of available SFPV and possible congenital duplication of the veins. More important, the ultrasound allows identification of deep venous thrombosis or recanalization, congenital absence of the SFPV, or preferential lower limb venous drainage through a dominant profunda femoral vein. Although not prohibitive, we consider these findings on duplex scan relative contraindications to removal of the SFPV. Imaging of both lower limbs should be performed because aberrant venous anatomy may be confined to a single limb with an entirely normal vein present in the contralateral limb. Venous mapping will also give information about the greater saphenous veins. These veins may be very useful if concomitant infrainguinal reconstruction is required after aortoiliac reconstruction.

The majority of our experience using this technique has been in the treatment of prosthetic aortic graft infection. We have not limited our reconstructions to patients with low-virulence prosthetic biofilm infections. In fact, we have treated a significant number of patients with polymicrobial infections with the infected graft sitting in a feculent abscess cavity. Previous cultures have grown in descending order of frequency: *Staphylococcus epidermidis, Staphylococcus aureus, Pseudomonas aeruginosa, Escherichia coli, Klebsiella* species, *Proprionibacterium acnes, Enterococcus faecalis, Enterobacter aerogenes, Streptococcus pyogenese, Bacteroides* species, *Acinetobacter bamanii, Salmonella* species, and *Mycobacterium tuberculosis*. Recently, several grafts have grown out fungal species. We have also applied the in situ aortic reconstruction with SFPV to patients requiring revascularization who have contraindications to prosthetic bypass because of regional infections, such as hydradenitis suppurativa and septic arteritis, and to patients with pan-infected axillofemoral grafts. A smaller number of patients have undergone autologous reconstruction in the absence of infection because of repeated failure of conventional prosthetic bypass, and in selected young patients as a primary procedure.

We have applied this technique in the treatment of aortic graft infection with aortoenteric fistula with mixed results. Initial experience with the technique in this subgroup of patients was unfavorable. Patients survived the procedure only to die in the postoperative period of multiple organ failure. These poor outcomes prompted our recommendations to avoid the use of this technique in patients with aortoenteric communications.[3]

SURGICAL TECHNIQUE

By necessity, the surgical treatment of infected aortic grafts and in situ reconstruction using SFPV requires a sequential single operation. As a result, the operations are of long duration, and are often associated with significant blood loss, metabolic derangement, and difficulty with core temperature control. Pulmonary artery catheters and transesophageal echocardiography are used routinely for intraoperative anesthesia monitoring. Fluids are given through blood warmers, and upper body heated air-warming blankets are used.

Two surgical teams usually work simultaneously to reduce overall operative time. One surgical team works to expose the infected aortic graft, while the other endeavors to expose the SFPVs. Surgical approaches are tailored to the clinical situation, but simultaneous lower extremity vein harvest and aortic graft dissection usually involves standard supine positioning and a transperitoneal approach to the abdominal aorta. However, we have also used the left flank retroperitoneal approach. If possible, we sequence the operation as follows: (1) dissect deep veins and leave in situ until needed; (2) isolate femoral vessels; (3) enter abdomen and obtain aortic control; (4) remove infected graft; and (5) perform reconstruction with SFPVs.

Positioning of the lower limbs requires external rotation at the hips and flexion at the knees. This "frog-leg" position is facilitated by a pillow placed on the operating table under the knees. Full aortic replacement will usually require bilateral vein harvest. Incisions are made over the lateral border of the sartorius muscle. In addition to allowing direct access to the contents of Hunter's canal, the lateral orientation of the incision anatomically isolates the wound from more medial infected femoral wounds. This approach also allows direct access to the more distal superficial femoral artery and profunda femoral artery beyond its primary branches. The sartorius muscle is reflected medially and posteriorly, allowing preservation of its medial segmental blood supply. The subsartorial canal is opened initially in the mid thigh. The superficial femoral artery is easily identified by gentle palpation and serves as a useful landmark for locating the neurovascular bundle. The superficial femoral artery is exposed along its anterior surface and the SFPV is readily identified posterior and medial to the artery. The saphenous nerve is intimately involved with the artery and vein and care must be taken during dissection to prevent injury; excessive traction or unplanned division will often result in an annoying postoperative medial leg neuralgia. Extreme care must be taken while mobilizing the branches of the superficial femoral artery, especially around the adductor hiatus. These branches may represent important collaterals to reconstituted distal arterial beds.

The SFPV has multiple side branches. These are double ligated and divided. The importance of secure branch ligature cannot be overemphasized. Exposure of the vein graft to aortic pressure will result in hemorrhage through poorly secured branch ligatures. The walls of the vein tend to become very thin near the insertion of side branches. Torn branches can be frustrating to repair because suture closure of the vein wall even with fine monofilament is difficult. It is best to avoid this with careful and patient dissection of all branches. Dissection is carried proximally to the confluence of the SFPV with the profunda femoral vein to form the common femoral vein. The profunda femoral vein is readily identified as a large-caliber vessel penetrating deep through the fascia constituting the floor of Hunter's canal. Distal dissection is facilitated by division of the adductor tendons to open the adductor hiatus. This allows easy access to the popliteal vein. The distal dissection at this level can be technically demanding; it is apparent from mutiple dissections at this level that the most side branches of the SFPV are found in the popliteal segment. When necessary, this vein can be exposed below the knee, adding an additional 10 cm of conduit. After complete mobilization of both SFPVs, the veins are left in situ until the required length of conduit can be determined. When ready for removal, the popliteal vein is divided and oversewn with a single suture ligature. The proximal SFPV is divided flush with the deep femoral vein and oversewn with a 5-0 nonabsorbable monofilament suture. This allows unimpeded flow from the profunda femoral vein to the common femoral vein and minimizes the possibility of thrombus forming in a residual venous cul-de-sac. The three or four large valves of the SFPV are easily identified and lysed using a valvulotome or directly excised by temporarily everting the vein graft. The nonreversed configuration will allow placement of the larger end of the vein at the proximal aortic anastomosis.

After removal of all infected prosthetic graft material and wide debridement of grossly infected aorta and surrounding soft tissues, selected revascularization to critical arterial beds is performed using the vein grafts. We have used several configurations of vein grafts based upon length of available conduit, degree of contamination, and other anatomic constraints, such as the presence of a left-sided diverticular abscess or a large psoas abscess (Fig 1). In addition, the surgeon must be able to adapt to different aortic sizes and size mismatch between the SFPV and the infrarenal aorta. We

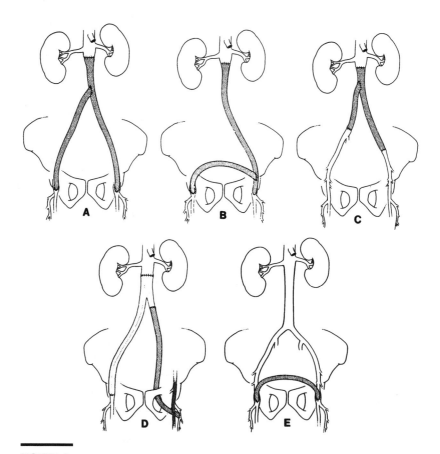

FIGURE 1.

Diagram depicts several configurations of aortic reconstruction using superficial femoral-popliteal vein grafts. Grafts are configured according to extent of infection, anatomical limitations, and length of available conduit.

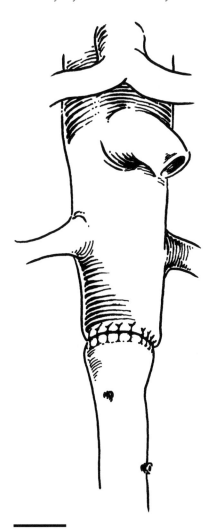

FIGURE 2.
A standard end-to-end aortic-vein graft anastomosis.

have used several proximal anastomotic variations (Figs 2–4). Although the diameters of the SFPV are fairly large (8–12 mm), anastomoses to 20-mm or greater diameter infrarenal aortic segments are frequently required. Despite moderate size mismatch, effective end-to-end anastomosis is possible with two-point or more fixation and careful suture placement to make up size discrepancies (Fig 2). Plication of the distal aorta may also be performed to reduce the diameter of the aorta at the anastomosis (Fig 3). If the size dis-

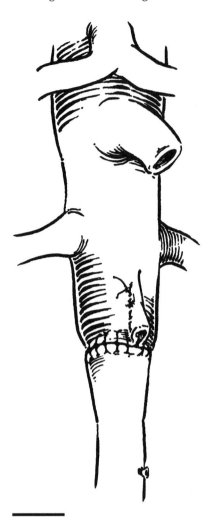

FIGURE 3.

Anterior aortic plication to reduce size mismatch between the infrarenal aorta and the vein graft.

crepancy results in an unreasonable size mismatch and if enough venous conduit is available, we also use a long pantaloon vein graft configuration (Fig 4). Use of this configuration has eliminated the problem of aortic-graft size mismatch at the proximal anastomosis, allowing the construction of end-to-end anastomoses with all infrarenal aortas.

After construction of the proximal anastomosis, the grafts are temporarily occluded and distended. This allows careful scrutiny of the vein graft side branches while subjected to aortic blood pres-

sure before tunneling. Proximal suture line bleeding should be repaired with the native aorta clamped to prevent tearing of the vein
graft during suture placement. If iliac anastomoses are required,
these are performed in a standard manner. Femoral graft limbs are
tunneled through the old debrided tunnels, or through new paral-

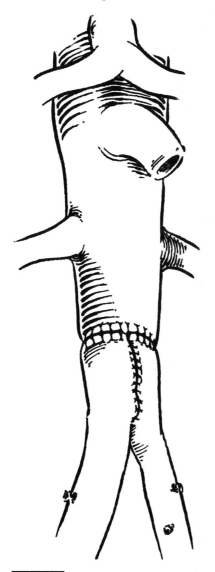

FIGURE 4.

An example of a proximal anastomosis with a pantaloon vein graft configuration.

lel noncontaminated tunnels. Care must be taken when pulling the vein grafts through the tunnels because side branch ligatures may be dislodged by excessive effort. To avoid this problem, we pass our vein grafts nondistended. Distal femoral anastomoses are performed using standard techniques. Occasionally, adjunctive profundaplasties or profunda reimplantation is required after extensive debridement of the common femoral artery and the femoral bifurcation after infected graft excision. This is especially true when dealing with large distal anastomotic false aneurysms where infection involves the femoral bifurcation. Particular care should be made to ensure some perfusion to the pelvis is provided in the form of retrograde blood flow from the groin to prevent pelvic, visceral, or spinal nerve root ischemia.

Assessment of distal limb perfusion before closure of wounds is essential. As mentioned earlier, when the superficial femoral arteries are occluded, inadvertent interruption of vital collaterals from the profunda femoral artery to the distal superficial femoral or popliteal arteries occurring during dissection of the SFPV can lead to leg ischemia, despite excellent inflow. In addition, acute venous hypertension in the leg combined with prolonged limb ischemia time during aortic reconstruction may lead to compartment syndromes. We have a low threshold for performing four-compartment leg fasciotomy to treat this problem. If Doppler flow does not improve after fasciotomy, infrainguinal reconstruction may be required as an adjunctive procedure to the aortoiliac reconstruction. For obvious reasons, we avoid the use of prosthetic material in concomitant infrainguinal bypass.

The wounds are all irrigated with antibiotic solution, and hemostasis is achieved. Drains are placed when appropriate. Wounds in infected fields are closed at the fascial level, but the skin is generally left open and packed with moist gauze. The vein harvest wounds are drained and closed in layers with absorbable suture and skin staples.

POSTOPERATIVE CARE

All patients are managed in the surgical ICU after the procedure. Fluid requirements are generally what one would expect from a major aortic operation. Antibiotics are modified as intraoperative culture results isolate specific organisms sensitive to specific antibiotic regimens. Intravenous antibiotics are stopped when the patient is clinically well, remains afebrile, and has a normal leukocyte count with a normal differential. This generally occurs 3–5 days after surgery. No long-term oral antibiotics are initiated.

We consider these patients to be at very high risk for developing postoperative venous thromboembolism. In the postoperative period, intermittent pneumatic compression plus low-dose subcutaneous heparin prophylaxis are used. The presumed stasis and intimal trauma in the residual popliteal vein mandates this aggressive approach. Virtually all patients have limited venous thrombosis in the residual popliteal vein "stump." Aggressive prophylaxis may prevent retrograde propagation into leg veins. We do not use long-term anticoagulation for this limited venous thrombosis; pulmonary embolism is unlikely because of the absence of the SFPV.

LONG-TERM FOLLOW-UP

Patients are seen every 3 months as an outpatient for the first year after surgery. Noninvasive vascular testing includes ankle-brachial pressure indices, photoplethysmographic toe pressures, aortoiliofemoral graft duplex examination, and venous studies. Surveillance is performed twice a year thereafter.

GRAFT PATENCY

We have found that these reconstructions are exceptionally durable. As we have previously reported,[3] with 37 grafts at risk and a mean follow-up of 32 ± 21 months, the primary patency was 83% at 5 years. Distal anastomotic intimal hyperplasia led to late graft failure in two patients. Both failures were treated successfully with anastomotic revision. Therefore, secondary graft patency at 5 years was 100%. These data are surprising given the degree of infrainguinal arterial occlusive disease present in this patient population. Using accepted "runoff scores" defined in the suggested reporting standards for reports dealing with lower extremity ischemia by the Joint Vascular Societies[4] in which a score of 1 indicates no distal disease below an anastomotic site, and a score of 10 indicates a blind vascular segment, the average "runoff score" in our cohort was 4.9 ± 2.6. In 68% of limbs, the profunda femoral or the superficial femoral artery was the sole runoff vessel.

In spite of the exposure of these thin-walled veins to aortic blood pressure, aneurysmal dilation of these grafts does not occur. Instead, our long-term graft surveillance has noted a slight decrease in diameter over time. The mean graft diameter at 6 months after implantation was 10.8 mm, compared with a diameter of 7.8 mm at 60 months.[3] In addition, no anastomotic dehiscences or anastomotic pseudoaneurysms have occurred, despite grafts placed in obviously infected beds. Anecdotally, we have examined several grafts explanted at autopsy of patients who have died of other medical causes months to years after in situ aortic grafting. Microscopic examination revealed a moderate amount of neointimal hyperplasia but with minimal lumen encroachment. We speculate that these arterialized veins develop a normal proliferative response, but because of their large caliber, these lesions rarely become hemodynamically significant.

SURVIVAL AND LIMB SALVAGE

As would be expected from a population with severe vascular disease, long-term survival has been poor. The majority have died of complications of coronary artery disease. The death rate for this group of patients has been approximately 10% per year. However, the amputation-free survival is considerably higher. In fact, the amputation-free survival roughly parallels graft patency, with more than 95% of patients free from amputation at 3 years.

VENOUS MORBIDITY

We maintain that removal of the SFPV is associated with relatively low morbidity. Venous hypertension is immediately evident after removal of the veins. Swelling and congestion of the legs are common but remain transient. Leg elevation and pneumatic compression will dramatically reduce the amount of swelling during the postoperative period. This rapid improvement in edema is typically seen in the days after mobilization of the excess total body water gained during the early postoperative period. Patients are discharged with antithrombotic thigh-high elastic stockings to help control edema that arises during prolonged ambulation. Regardless of the presence or absence of a greater saphenous vein ipsilateral to a deep vein harvest site, lower limb swelling typically resolves completely after 6–8 weeks. There have been no cases of late venous claudication, stasis dermatitis, or venous stasis ulceration in any patient.

Our studies of venous physiology in the noninvasive laboratory using duplex ultrasound with rapid cuff deflation, venous refill times, and venous plethysmography all demonstrate evidence of significant venous outflow obstruction. However, the profunda femoral vein becomes the major outflow vessel of the lower limb. Large collateral veins are readily seen in the popliteal fossa communicating with the distal profunda femoral vein. Our findings confirm the observation of others[5–8] who have found a paucity of symptoms of chronic venous insufficiency associated with removal or ligation of the SFPV. We should caution that venous morbidity may require decades to develop, and our relatively brief average follow-up of 3 years is insufficient time to prove the relative benignity of deep vein harvest.

DISCUSSION

The accepted treatment of aortic graft infection is excision of the infected prosthesis and restoration of lower extremity blood flow. Revascularization after graft excision is usually established by extra anatomic bypass, with axillofemoral bypass being the long-standing preferred method of bypass. Despite the relative simplicity of this therapeutic strategy, patients treated for aortic graft infection continue to have significant morbidity, mortality, and limb loss. Investigators have reported operative mortality of 14% to 28%, and limb loss rates approaching 30%.[9–13] Without question, these patients are medically ill. Comorbid coronary, renal, and pulmonary disease, combined with the metabolic stress associated with chronic infection, place these patients at higher risk for operative complications and death. The stress associated with reoperative aortic surgery and graft excision undoubtedly contributes to operative morbidity. Notwithstanding, outcomes have been improved by staged revascularization followed by aortic graft excision, improvements in anesthesia and surgical critical care, and externally supported prosthetic grafts for long extra anatomic bypasses.[10, 11, 14] As a result, modern series examining the strategy of extra anatomic bypass and aortic graft excision report acceptable operative mortality and morbidity.[15] In addition to these unavoidable problems, compromised patency and secondary graft infection also add to late morbidity and limb loss associated with axillofemoral bypass placed for aortic graft infection.[10, 11, 13] The rate of secondary infection of axillofemoral bypass ranges from 13% to 27%.[10, 11, 13] Failure of these grafts secondary to infection is associated with tremendous morbidity and significant limb loss.[13, 16]

Our preference for in situ aortic reconstruction with SFPV is largely based upon the poor long-term performance of axillofemoral bypass for revascularization after removal of infected aortic grafts. The use of autologous conduits for revascularization after aortic graft excision is not new. In 1979, Ehrenfeld and colleagues[17] reported a series of 24 patients with graft infection, 15 with aortofemoral graft infection, treated with autologous reconstructions using endarterectomized superficial femoral arteries, greater saphenous veins, or composite prosthetic-autologous conduits. The authors noted no suture line dehiscences in infrarenal aortic-autologous graft anastomoses placed in infected fields; the maintenance of aortic continuity after graft excision seemed to avoid the risk of aortic stump disruption. These observations have been confirmed by other investigators examining the short-term utility of autologous reconstruction in the aortofemoral position or for femoral-femoral bypass for unilateral groin infection.[1, 18–20] Unfortunately, greater saphenous veins are technically difficult to use; kinking, twisting, and size mismatch are frequently encountered problems. In addition, many develop extensive neointimal hyperplasia, leading to a significant reduction in long-term graft patency.

As an alternative to greater saphenous vein and endarterectomized superficial femoral artery conduits, other authors have investigated the use of aortic homografts for in situ aortic replacement after graft excision.[21, 22] Kieffer et al.[21] used aortic homografts to treat 43 patients with infected infrarenal aortic prostheses. Postoperative mortality in the series was 12%, including death resulting from proximal aortic anastomotic dehiscence in a single patient. Four early graft-related complications occurred in three patients: early thrombosis, two episodes of septic graft rupture, and a graft-enteric fistula. Late graft-related complications occurred in 25% of survivors, the majority related to late stenoses secondary to chronic rejection. Two patients had aneurysmal degeneration of their allografts. In addition to the problems of reduced graft longevity, graft procurement from cadaver donors necessitated graft implantation in a recipient within 21 days to prevent late degenerative changes. The more recent experience of Vogt and associates [22] utilized cryopreserved aortic homografts in the treatment of aortic infections. Although applied to treatment of a variety of aortic infections, the authors reported 12 patients with infrarenal aortic infection. Despite a relatively brief follow-up period (18 months), their results were admirable.

Since our initial experience with in situ autologous aortic reconstruction using SFPV was reported in 1993, we have used this technique with increasing enthusiasm as an effective, safe, and durable means of treating aortic graft infection.[1] Others have independently achieved results equal to our own in many ways.[23] Nevelsteen and colleagues[23] reported their experience using the SFPV in similar patients in 1994. They performed in situ aortic reconstruction using SFPV in 15 patients with infrarenal aortoiliofemoral graft infections. Their operative mortality of 7% was admirable. Graft patency was 100% at a mean follow-up of 17 months. Amputation-free survival was comparable to our own experience.

SUMMARY

Autogenous aortoiliofemoral reconstruction using SFPV is a durable and successful means of treating aortic graft infection. The SFPV grafts resist gram-positive, gram-negative, and fungal infections. Superficial femoral-popliteal vein reconstruction allows eradication of infection while minimizing the risk of secondary graft infection. Maintenance of aortic continuity with an aortic-autograft anastomosis prevents the problem of aortic stump dehiscence. In addition, these reconstructions provide excellent long-term patency without aneurysmal deterioration or excessive neointimal hyperplasia, even in the setting of compromised run-off. Limb salvage rates are correspondingly high, and late venous morbidity is minimal.

REFERENCES

1. Clagett GP, Bowers BL, Lopez-Viego MA, et al: Creation of a neo-aortoiliac system from lower extremity deep and superficial veins. *Ann Surg* 218:239–249, 1993.
2. Hagino RT, Bengtson TD, Fosdick DA, et al: Venous reconstructions using the superficial femoral-popliteal vein. *J Vasc Surg* 26:829–837, 1997.
3. Clagett GP, Valentine RJ, Hagino RT: Autogenous aortoiliac/femoral reconstruction from superficial femoral-popliteal veins: Feasibility and durability. *J Vasc Surg* 25:255–270, 1997.
4. Rutherford RB, Flanigan DP, Gupta SK, et al: Suggested standards for reports dealing with lower extremity ischemia. *J Vasc Surg* 4:80–94, 1986.
5. Schulman ML, Badhey MR, Yatco R: Superficial femoral-popliteal veins and reversed saphenous veins as primary femoropopliteal bypass grafts: A randomized comparative study. *J Vasc Surg* 6:1–10, 1987.
6. Schanzer H, Chiang K, Mabrouk M, et al: Use of lower extremity deep veins as arterial substitutes: Functional status of the donor leg. *J Vasc Surg* 14:624–627, 1991.
7. Sladen JG, Downs AR: Superficial femoral vein. *Semin Vasc Surg* 8:209–215, 1995.
8. Masuda EM, Kistner RL, Ferris EB III: Long-term effects of superficial femoral vein ligation: Thirteen year follow-up. *J Vasc Surg* 16:741–749, 1992.
9. Reilly LM, Altman H, Lusby RJ, et al: Late results following surgical management of vascular graft infection. *J Vasc Surg* 1:36–44, 1984.
10. Reilly LM, Stoney RJ, Goldstone J, et al: Improved management of aortic graft infection: The influence of operation sequence and staging. *J Vasc Surg* 5:421–431, 1987.

11. O'Hara PJ, Hertzer NM, Beven EG, et al: Surgical management of infected abdominal aortic grafts: Review of a 25-year experience. *J Vasc Surg* 3:725–731, 1986.
12. Ricotta JJ, Faggioli GL, Stella A, et al: Total excision and extra-anatomic bypass for aortic graft infection. *Am J Surg* 162:145–149, 1991.
13. Yeager RA, Moneta GL, Taylor LM, et al: Improving survival and limb salvage in patients with aortic graft infection. *Am J Surg* 159:466–469, 1990.
14. Harris EJ, Taylor LM, McConnell DB, et al: Clinical results of axillo-bifemoral bypass using externally supported polytetrafluoroethylene. *J Vasc Surg* 12:416–421, 1990.
15. Sharp WJ, Hoballah JJ, Mohan CR, et al: The management of the infected aortic prosthesis: A current decade of experience. *J Vasc Surg* 19:844–850, 1994.
16. De Virgilio C, Cherry KJ, Gloviczki P, et al: Infected lower extremity extra-anatomic bypass grafts: Management of a serious complication in high-risk patients. *Ann Vasc Surg* 9:459–466 1995.
17. Ehrenfeld WK, Wilbur BG, Olcott CN, et al: Autogenous tissue reconstruction in the management of infected prosthetic grafts. *Surgery* 85:82–92, 1979.
18. Lorentzen JE, Nielsen OM: Aortobifemoral bypass with autogenous saphenous vein in the treatment of paninfected aortic bifurcation graft. *J Vasc Surg* 3:666–668, 1986.
19. Seeger JM, Wheeler JR, Gregory RT, et al: Autogenous graft replacement of infected prosthetic grafts in the femoral position. *Surgery* 93:39–45, 1983.
20. Jicha DL, Reilly LM, Kuestner LM, et al: Durability of cross-femoral grafts after aortic graft infection: The fate of autogenous conduits. *J Vasc Surg* 22:393–407, 1995.
21. Kieffer E, Bahnini A, Koskas F, et al: In situ allograft replacement of infected infrarenal aortic prosthetic grafts: Results in forty-three patients. *J Vasc Surg* 17:349–356, 1993.
22. Vogt PR, Segesser LK, Goffin Y, et al: Eradication of aortic infections with the use of cryopreserved arterial homografts. *Ann Thorac Surg* 62:640–645, 1996.
23. Nevelsteen A, Lacroix H, Suy R: Autogenous reconstruction with the lower extremity deep veins: An alternative treatment of prosthetic infections after reconstructive surgery for aortoiliac disease. *J Vasc Surg* 22:129–134, 1995.

CHAPTER 4

Update Regarding Current Utility of Endoluminal Prostheses for Aortoiliac Disease

Michael L. Marin, M.D.
Associate Professor of Surgery, Mount Sinai School of Medicine, Director, Endovascular Surgical Development, The Mount Sinai Medical Center, New York, New York

Larry H. Hollier, M.D.
Julius H. Jacobson II, M.D., Professor of Vascular Surgery, Chairman, Department of Surgery, Mount Sinai School of Medicine, Surgeon in Chief, The Mount Sinai Medical Center, New York, New York

Harold A. Mitty, M.D.
Professor of Radiology, Mount Sinai School of Medicine, Attending Radiologist, The Mount Sinai Medical Center, New York, New York

Richard Parsons, M.D.
Assistant Professor of Surgery, Mount Sinai School of Medicine, The Mount Sinai Medical Center, New York, New York

James M. Cooper, M.D.
Assistant Professor of Radiology, Mount Sinai School of Medicine, Attending Radiologist, The Mount Sinai Medical Center, New York, New York

T he endovascular treatment of aortoiliac disease continues to evolve. Iliac angioplasty with intravascular stent support has become a widely accepted treatment for symptomatic focal lesions of the common iliac arteries.[1-3] More extensive occlusive disease of the aortoiliac segment has also been approached with balloon angioplasty and stenting techniques with less favorable results.[4, 5] Long-segment occlusive disease or aneurysmal lesions have, until recently, been excluded from treatments that use minimally inva-

Advances in Vascular Surgery®, vol. 6
© 1998, Mosby, Inc.

sive catheter-based technologies. The evolution of new devices that blend stent and prosthetic graft technologies is beginning to take form in the treatment of arterial aneurysm, occlusion, and trauma. This chapter will explore the application of these devices to the treatment of the various pathologies affecting the aorta and iliac vessels.

ENDOGRAFTS FOR ANEURYSMS

The use of endovascular grafts for aneurysmal disease continues to be one of the most challenging applications of this technology since its original introduction by Parodi et al. in 1990.[6] Achieving a water-tight seal between the graft and the aortic wall remains one of the more complex challenges of the devices presently in clinical use.[7, 8] Currently, aortoiliac aneurysms are being treated by one of three endovascular grafting techniques. Aorto-bifemoral endografts constructed from single prostheses were originally described by Chuter et al. and are the basis for the current clinical trials being performed by the Endovascular Technologies Corporation (Menlo-Park, Calif).[9, 10] This endograft design is inserted into the vascular system through one iliofemoral system, and the contralateral limb of a bifurcated graft is advanced into positioning by means of a cross-femoral wire (Fig 1). Great care must be exercised to avoid twisting of the contralateral iliac limb as it is being advanced to its final position. Results using this technique on 52 patients have been reported by Chuter et al.; the procedure success rate was 94%, the endoleak rate was 11%, and the mortality rate was 2% with follow-up to 3 years.[11]

The second approach to aortoiliac aneurysms is an aorto-uni-iliac graft, contralateral common iliac artery occlusion, and a standard femoral-to-femoral crossover bypass. This approach was initially described by Parodi and has been adopted by several centers around the world.[12–15] After the insertion of a tapered endograft from the infrarenal aorta to the iliac or femoral artery, an occlusion device is inserted into the contralateral common iliac artery to prevent retrograde flow into the aneurysm sac. The reconstruction is completed by placing a standard femorofemoral bypass in a subcutaneous suprapubic tunnel (Fig 2). This approach is particularly useful for treating complex, highly tortuous aneurysms.

The final approach in current clinical practice for treating aortoiliac aneurysms uses variations of a "modular" device. This system is composed of a number of pieces that can be "mixed and

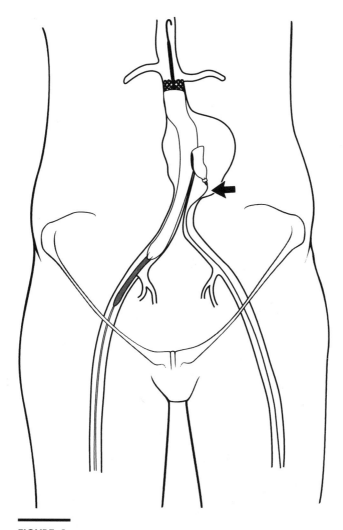

FIGURE 1.

Schematic drawing of a single-piece aortic endovascular graft. Both iliac graft limbs are inserted together in one delivery sheath, and one limb is advanced into position by means of traction on a cross-femoral wire *(arrow)*.

matched" and assembled in situ to achieve some variation in device length. Many devices in clinical trials (Vanguard, Meadox Medical; Aneurx, Medtronics; Excluder, Prograft Medical; TALENT, World Medical) use this design with a main aortic body section into which extending iliac limbs are inserted (Fig 3). Initial experience with the Vanguard modular system has been favorable.

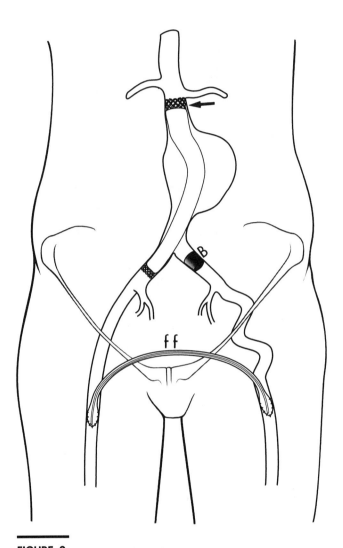

FIGURE 2.

Schematic drawing of an aorto-ilio-femoral bypass. This configuration is the simplest to construct and is quite versatile with respect to complex aortoiliac anatomy. The endograft is inserted through a single common femoral artery and fixed to the pararenal aortic neck by means of a stent *(arrow)*. This distal end of the endograft is tacked to the distal common iliac artery by means of a stent. A covered stent that has been tied off distally like a "wind sock" is deployed into the contralateral common iliac artery to prevent retrograde flow into the aneurysm sac *(B)*. A conventional femorofemoral bypass completes the reconstruction *(ff)*.

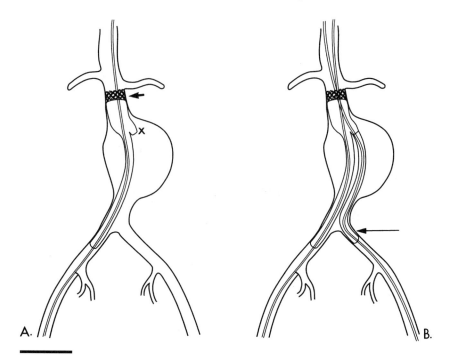

FIGURE 3.

Schematic drawing of a "modular" endovascular grafting system for repair of an abdominal aortic aneurysm. **A,** the main body of the device is inserted into the ipsilateral common femoral artery and advanced and deployed at the level of the pararenal aortic neck *(arrow)* x = short limb. **B,** after recanalizing a contralateral short iliac limb with a guidewire, a graft extension is inserted to connect the contralateral iliac prosthesis into position in the common iliac artery *(arrow)*.

Blum et al. described 149 patients who had an 89% success rate, which included 13% endoleaks, 3% conversion to open repair, and a 1% mortality rate during 13 months of follow-up.[16]

Aneurysms localized to the iliac arteries may also be treated by endovascular grafts that are designed to accommodate the underlying pathology (Fig 4).[17] These lesions have a variable morphology that often require a combination of endovascular techniques (endograft insertions, occlusion coils) and local open surgical procedures (vascular access, endograft end-point customization). Several different devices have been successfully used to treat isolated iliac aneurysms, including Palmaz-based, balloon-expandable stent-based grafts as well as self-expanding systems constructed from Nitinol Metalanol fabric (Passager, Meadox Medical/Boston Scientific, Oakland, NJ) (Fig 5).[18, 19]

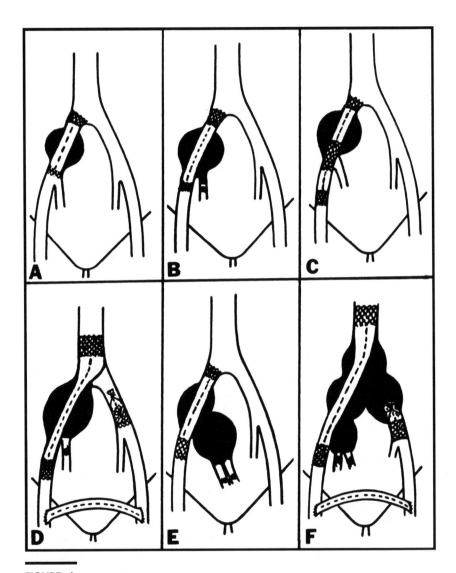

FIGURE 4.
Schematic drawing of the various ways to repair isolated common iliac artery aneurysms. (Courtesy of Marin ML, Veith FJ, Lyon R: Transfemoral endovascular repair of iliac artery aneurysm. *Am J Surg* 170:179–182. Copyright 1995 by Excerpta Medica Inc. Reprinted with permission.)

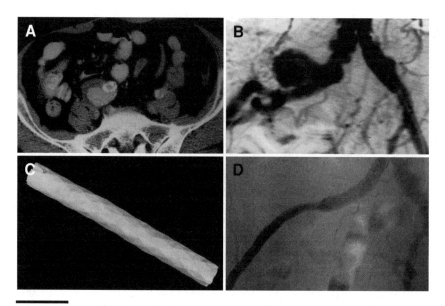

FIGURE 5.

Endoluminal repair of a ruptured common iliac artery aneurysm. **A,** CT scan of a patient with the acute onset of back pain before demonstrating a common iliac aneurysm with contrast extending beyond the confines of the vessel wall. **B,** angiogram of the contained rupture of a right common iliac aneurysm before repair. **C,** photograph of a Passager self-expanding endovascular graft. This Nitinol-based device expands to its final form after insertion into the vessel. **D,** angiogram after insertion of the endograft demonstrating exclusion of the aneurysm.

ENDOGRAFTS FOR OCCLUSIVE AORTOILIAC DISEASE

Occlusive aortoiliac disease has been an important application of endovascular graft procedures, bridging the shortcomings of intravascular stent and bypass graft technologies. Long-segment disease appears to be ideal for this procedure, allowing for less invasive treatments of symptomatic patients (Fig 6).[19–21] Primary and secondary patency for long aortoiliac stenoses or occlusions have been favorable, ranging between 80% to 89% and 100%, respectively. Limb salvage in a group of medically high-risk patients was between 94% and 100%.[20, 21]

ENDOVASCULAR GRAFTS FOR PSEUDOANEURYSM AND TRAUMA

The use of endovascular grafts for the treatment of trauma represents one of the most important advances in the treatment of these complex lesions. Focal injuries to medium-sized arteries (subclavian, femoral) have been successfully treated using non–

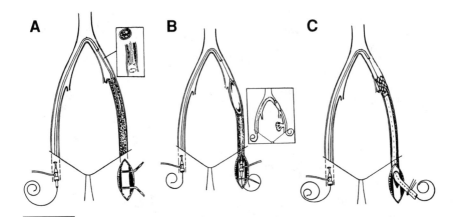

FIGURE 6.

Schematic drawing of an approach to endoluminal repair of iliac artery occlusive disease. **A,** the long segment occluded left external iliac artery is recanalized percutaneously by a contralateral approach. **B,** the entire occluded segment of the vessel is balloon dilated to create a tract for inserting the new endograft. **C,** after deployment of the aortoiliac stent graft, aortic inflow is reestablished by anastomosis to the most suitable outflow vessel. (Courtesy of Marin ML, Veith FJ, Sanchez LA et al: Endovascular aortoiliac grafts in combination with standard infrainguinal arterial bypasses in the management of limb-threatening ischemia: Preliminary report. *J Vasc Surg* 22:316–325, 1995. Reprinted with permission.)

porous-covered stent devices.[22] Treatment of pseudoaneurysm and trauma of the aortoiliac segment includes penetrating injuries to vessels, ruptured aneurysms, and para-anastomotic lesions caused by either a breakdown of a standard repair or progression of vascular disease with a deterioration of the vessel wall.[22–24] The principles of endovascular treatment of these lesions is analogous to conventional reconstruction techniques, namely, a repair (endograft) must extend from healthy tissue above to below the lesion (Fig 7). Based on our experience with traumatic pseudoaneurysms and para-anastomotic lesions, endovascular grafts may rapidly become the primary treatment of these difficult clinical problems.[20, 24] The ability to repair an arterial segment from a remote site without dissecting within a traumatized field or redissecting a scarred previous reconstruction area is one of the most important advantages of these new devices and techniques.

SUMMARY

Endovascular grafts continue to evolve with regard to device structure, procedure detail, and clinical application. The use of these devices to repair arterial aneurysms, occlusions, and trauma of the

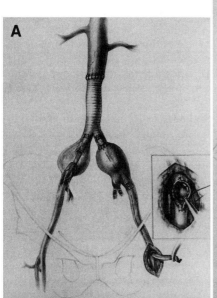
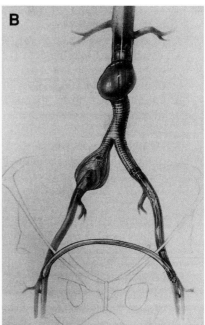

FIGURE 7.

Endoluminal grafts for treating para-anastomotic aneurysm. **A,** schematic drawing of simple tubular endograft designs for repairing both true *(left)* and false *(right)* aorto-iliac aneurysms. The grafts may be extended to the common femoral artery where an endoluminal anastomosis is created **(inset). B,** more complex lesions may be bridged with an aorto-uni-iliac-femoral-femoral reconstruction. (Courtesy of Yuan JG, Marin ML, Veith FJ, et al: Endovascular grafts for non-infected aortoiliac anastomotic aneurysm. *J Vasc Surg* 26:210–221, 1997. Reprinted with permission.)

aortoiliac segment has achieved favorable early results. Long-term follow-up with an eye on the durability of repair and procedure-related complications is essential in evaluating the true impact of these less-invasive devices on vascular disease management.

REFERENCES

1. Johnston KW: Iliac arteries: Reanalysis of results of balloon angioplasty. *Radiology* 186:207–212, 1993.
2. Palmaz JC, Laborde JC, Rivera FJ, et al: Stenting of the iliac arteries with the Palmaz stent: Experience from a multicenter trial. *Cardiovasc Intervent Radiol* 15:291–297, 1992.
3. Bosch JL, Hunink MG: Meta-analysis of the results of percutaneous transluminal angioplasty and stent placement for aortoiliac occlusive disease. *Radiology* 204:87–96, 1997.

4. Laborde JC, Palmaz JC, Rivera FJ, et al: Influence of anatomic distribution of atherosclerosis on the outcome of revascularization with iliac stent placement. *J Vasc Interv Radiol* 6:513–521, 1995.
5. Vorwerk D, Guenther RW, Schurmann K, et al: Primary stent placement for chronic iliac artery occlusions: Follow-up results in 103 patients. *Radiology* 194:745–749, 1995.
6. Parodi JC, Palmaz JC, Barone HD: Transfemoral intravascular graft implantation for abdominal aortic aneurysm. *Ann Vasc Surg* 5:491–499, 1991.
7. White GH, Yu W, May J, et al: Endoleak as a complication of endoluminal grafting of abdominal aortic aneurysm: Classification, incidence, diagnosis and management. *J Endovasc Surg* 4:152–168, 1997.
8. Wain RA, Marin ML, Ohki T, et al: Endoleaks complicating endovascular graft treatment of aortic aneurysm: Classification, risk factors and outcome. *J Vasc Surg,* 27:69–80, 1998.
9. Chuter TAM, Green RM, Ouriel K, et al: Transfemoral endovascular aortic graft placement. *J Vasc Surg* 18:185–197, 1993.
10. Edwards WH, Naslund T, Edwards WH, et al: Endovascular grafting of abdominal aortic aneurysms: A preliminary study. *Ann Surg* 223:568–575, 1996.
11. Chuter TAM, Wendt G, Hopkinson BR, et al: European experience with a system for bifurcated stent-graft insertion. *J Endovasc Surg* 4:13–22, 1997.
12. Parodi JC: Endovascular repair of aortic aneurysm, arteriovenous fistulas and false aneurysm. *World J Surg* 20:655–663, 1996.
13. Marin ML, Veith FJ, Cynamon J, et al: Initial experience with transitionally placed endovascular grafts for the treatment of complex vascular lesions. *Ann Surg* 222:449–469, 1995.
14. Yusef SW, Whitaker SC, Chuter TAM: Early results of endovascular aortic aneurysm surgery with aortouniiliac graft, contralateral iliac occlusions, and femorofemoral bypass. *J Vasc Surg* 25:165–172, 1997.
15. Kato N, Dake MD, Semba CP, et al: Treatment of aortoiliac aneurysm with use of a single-piece tapered stent graft. *JVIR* 9:41–49, 1998.
16. Blum V, Voshage G, Beyersdorf F, et al: Two center German experience with aortic endografting. *J Endovasc Surg* 4:137–146, 1997.
17. Marin ML, Veith FJ, Lyon R: Transfemoral endovascular repair of iliac artery aneurysm. *Am J Surg* 170:179–182, 1995.
18. Parsons R, Marin ML, Hollier LH: Midterm experience with endovascular grafts to treat isolated common iliac artery aneurysm. *J Vasc Surg,* in press.
19. Amor M, Henry M: Role of covered stents in the interventional percutaneous treatment of peripheral aneurysms. International Symposium on Vascular Diagnosis and Intervention. Miami, Fla, January 1998.
20. Marin ML, Veith FJ, Sanchez LA, et al: Endovascular repair of aortoiliac occlusive disease. *World J Surg* 20:679–686, 1996.

21. Henry M, Amor M, Henry I, et al: Endoluminal bypass grafting in leg arteries with the Cragg Endopro System I: A series of 105 patients. *J Endovasc Surg* 3:118, 1996.
22. Marin ML, Veith FJ, Panetta TF, et al: Transluminally placed endovascular stented grafts for repair of arterial trauma. *J Vasc Surg* 20:466–473, 1994.
23. Yusuf SW, Whitaker SC, Chuter TAM, et al: Emergency endovascular repair of leaking aortic aneurysm. *Lancet* 344:1645, 1994.
24. Yuan JG, Marin ML, Veith FJ, et al: Endovascular grafts for non-infected aortoiliac anastomotic aneurysms. *J Vasc Surg* 26:210–221, 1997.

CHAPTER 5

Endoleak—A Complication Unique to Endovascular Grafting: The Sydney Experience

James May, M.S., F.R.A.C.S., F.A.C.S.
Bosch Professor of Surgery, Department of Surgery, University of Sydney; Attending Surgeon, Department of Vascular Surgery, Royal Prince Alfred Hospital, Sydney, New South Wales, Australia

Geoffrey H. White, M.S., F.R.A.C.S.
Clinical Associate Professor of Surgery, Department of Surgery, University of Sydney; Attending Surgeon, Department of Vascular Surgery, Royal Prince Alfred Hospital, Sydney, New South Wales, Australia

T he endoluminal method of aneurysm repair has proven to be a much less invasive method than the conventional open operation. Blood loss at operation, the need for postoperative intensive care, and length of hospital stay are significantly less with the endoluminal technique.[1] The major limiting factors with endoluminal aneurysm repair are an unknown long-term outcome and a high rate of local/vascular complications. Improvements in technology have produced smaller diameter and more flexible delivery systems, which have reduced the incidence of damage to iliac arteries. Failure to isolate the aneurysm from the general circulation, however, remains a cause for concern. Such failure is likely to result in a further expansion of the aneurysm sac with the potential for rupture.

NOMENCLATURE

Failure to isolate the aneurysm from the circulation may be detected by angiography, CT, or duplex ultrasound imaging. This phenomenon has been described in the early literature on endoluminal aneurysm repair as a "leak." This term, however, is confusing because it has been common practice to use the word "leak" to refer to extravasation of blood outside the aorta associated with aneurysm rupture. We proposed that a more specific term for failure to exclude the aneurysm from the circulation would be "endoleak."[2] This term would be unique to endoluminal grafts because the leak of blood remains within the confines of the vessel but external to the endoluminal graft. We suggested the following definition of endoleak:

> Endoleak is a condition associated with endoluminal vascular grafts, defined by the persistence of blood flow outside the lumen of the endoluminal graft but within an aneurysm sac or adjacent vascular segment being treated by the graft. Endoleak is due to incomplete sealing or exclusion of the aneurysm sac or vessel segment as evidenced by imaging studies such as contrast-enhanced CT, ultrasonography, or angiography.[3]

CLASSIFICATION OF ENDOLEAK BY TYPE

We further proposed that a clear distinction should be made between endoleak related to the graft device itself and endoleak associated with flow from collateral arterial branches.[4] We proposed that these be identified as being either type 1 or type 2 endoleak as classified by the following system.

TYPE 1 ENDOLEAK (GRAFT-RELATED ENDOLEAK)

Type 1 endoleak occurs when a persistent channel of blood flow develops because of an inadequate or ineffective seal at the graft ends (or between segments of overlapping graft segments). It can usually be determined whether this is at the proximal, midgraft, or distal graft aspects, and these qualifiers should be added. Endoleak at the midgraft region may be caused by leakage through a defect in the graft fabric, or may be between segments of a modular multisegment graft (Fig 1).

TYPE 2 ENDOLEAK (NON–GRAFT-RELATED ENDOLEAK)

Type 2 endoleak occurs when there is persistent collateral blood flow into the aneurysm sac flowing retrogradely from patent lumbar arteries, the inferior mesenteric artery, the intercostal arteries (in thoracic aneurysms), or other collateral vessels. In this situation there is usually a complete seal around the graft attachment zones so that the complication is not related directly to the graft itself.

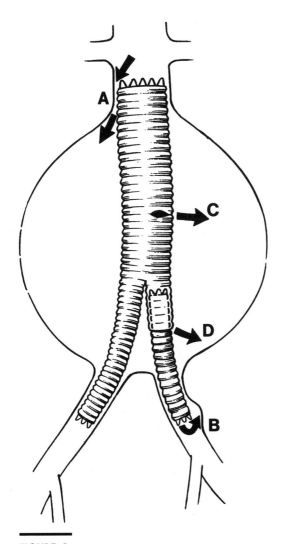

FIGURE 1.

Endoleak associated with endovascular grafts may occur: proximally *(A)*; distally from the graft limbs in the iliac arteries *(B)*; at the midgraft region *(C)*; or between the segments of a modular graft *(D)*. (Reproduced with permission from *J Endovasc Surg*).

CLASSIFICATION OF ENDOLEAK BY TIME OF OCCURRENCE

In addition to classification by type, endoleak may also be classified according to when it occurs.

PRIMARY ENDOLEAK

Primary endoleak is present from the time of the implantation procedure, or is initially diagnosed during the 30-day perioperative period.

SECONDARY ENDOLEAK (OR LATE ENDOLEAK)

Secondary endoleak occurs as a late event after a successful endoluminal graft implantation procedure. No endoleak is present at the time of implantation or during the perioperative period.

RECURRENT ENDOLEAK

Recurrent endoleak has been demonstrated to have sealed spontaneously, then recurred subsequently.

ETIOLOGY OF ENDOLEAK

Patient selection and sizing of an endograft based on pre-operative imaging are important determinants in the risk of developing an endoleak. The morphology of the aorta and aneurysm is clearly related to this risk also. There is general agreement on the following criteria for using the endoluminal method: that proximal neck of an abdominal aortic aneurysm (AAA) should be 15 mm in length or greater and 26 mm in diameter or less. Angulation, calcification and mural thrombus in the neck also increase the risk of endoleak. The etiology of endoleak is summarized in Table 1. These features are usually responsible for primary endoleak. Secondary or late endoleak, however, is becoming a major long-term complication of the endoluminal method. This may result from displacement of the proximal or distal ends of the endograft or distraction of component parts of a modular graft.

INCIDENCE AND NATURAL HISTORY OF ENDOLEAK

The incidence of endoleak has been variously reported at 44% by Moore and Rutherford,[5] 27% by Marin et al.,[6] and 10% or less by Blum et al.,[7] Parodi,[8] and May et al.[9]

Untreated, an endoleak leads to continued expansion of the AAA.[10-12] The endoleak may seal spontaneously by thrombosis. This occurred in more than half the cases of endoleak reported by Moore and Rutherford, leaving them with a permanent endoleak rate of 21%. Spontaneous sealing of the endoleak is accompanied

TABLE 1.
Etiology of Endoleak

Graft Related
   Problems in Graft Sizing or Patient Selection
      Graft size mismatch (length/diameter)
      Graft overlap zone mismatch (length/diameter)
      Mismatch of graft shape to aortic morphology (e.g., rigid stent in
         angulated aneurysm neck)
   Unfavorable Aortic Morphology
      Short neck or attachment zone
      Angulated neck or irregular lumen shape
   Graft Damage
      Graft tear/fragile graft fabric
      Graft tear/suture damage to graft fabric
      Graft perforation due to guidewire
      Graft dilatation
      Balloon or sheath trauma to graft
   Implantation Technique Problems
      Graft misplacement
      Graft displacement
      Incomplete graft expansion
Non–Graft Related
      Large Patent Lumbar Arteries
      Large Patent Inferior Mesenteric Artery
      Large Patent Intercostal Arteries (Thoracic Endograft)
      Other Collateral Flow

by reduction in the diameter of the AAA (Fig 2). Conversely, the diameter of the AAA increases when a secondary endoleak develops in a previously isolated AAA after successful endoluminal repair.

In reviewing an extensive series of endoluminal AAA repairs using EVT (Endovascular Technologies, Menlo Park, California) prostheses, Bernhard[13] reported that type 2 endoleaks were more likely to seal spontaneously than type 1. It has also been suggested that type 2 endoleaks may be less likely to rupture. This may be a dangerous supposition, however, because the Albany group[14] has reported rupture of an AAA caused by collateral channels in patients treated by ligation and bypass. Untreated endoleak (type 1) resulting in AAA rupture has now been reported on three occasions.[8, 15, 16]

RELATIONSHIP OF AAA DIAMETER AND COMMUNICATION BETWEEN THE ANEURYSMAL SAC AND THE CIRCULATION IN FIVE PATIENTS

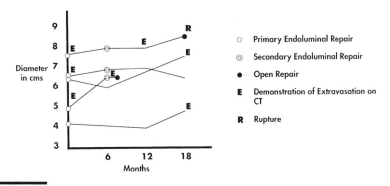

FIGURE 2.

Graph demonstrating increase in diameter following perioperative extravasation of contrast in 3 patients. No further increase was noted in 2 of these following secondary endoluminal repair until extravasation was again noted in 1. In the remaining 2 patients extravasation was not noted until 18 months after operation. This was preceded by a period of diminution in AAA diameter followed by an increase in diameter exceeding the preoperative figure. (Reproduced with permission from *Eur J Vasc Endovasc Surg*).

DIAGNOSIS OF ENDOLEAK

Physical examination of patients undergoing successful endoluminal repair of AAA usually reveals a nonexpansile mass or no mass, depending on the size of the aneurysm before treatment. Conversely, a presumptive diagnosis of endoleak may be made after endoluminal repair if the aneurysm is still found to have an expansile pulsation more than 48 hours after operation. This, however, is not an infallible test because it is possible for a pulsation to be transmitted through liquid thrombus.

Primary endoleak may be first detected by on-table postprocedure angiography. It is important that a power injector be used with cine-loop angiography with the capability of digital subtraction and frame-by-frame replay. It is also important that the angiographic catheter be placed at three levels: (1) at the level of the renal arteries near the proximal end of the graft; (2) at the midsection of the graft; and (3) distal to the graft, to check for perigraft reflux that may not have been detected on previous films.

INTRAOPERATIVE PRESSURE MEASUREMENTS

Intraoperative pressure measurements taken from a fine arterial catheter positioned within the aneurysm sac via the femoral artery have been recommended as a means of determining successful exclusion of the sac from the general circulation[17] (Fig 3). Exclusion is accompanied by a drop in systolic pressure and a dampening of

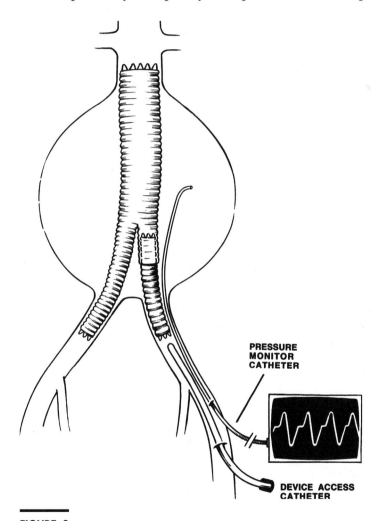

FIGURE 3

A 4F catheter is positioned percutaneously into the aneurysm via an iliac artery for monitoring pressure changes within the sac during endograft implantation. (Reproduced with permission from *J Endovasc Surg*).

the pressure wave. Harris,[18] however, has pointed out that despite these changes, the mean arterial pressure within the aneurysm sac remains unchanged for 24 hours after graft deployment.

CONTRAST-ENHANCED CT
It is advisable to perform contrast-enhanced CT within the first week after endoluminal repair. Endoleak is diagnosed by the presence of contrast outside the lumen of the endoluminal graft but within the lumen of the aneurysm sac (Fig 4). This method of imaging is considered to be more sensitive than angiography and may detect an endoleak unsuspected at operation.[19]

DUPLEX ULTRASOUND IMAGING
Despite increasing support for this noninvasive method of monitoring patients after endoluminal AAA repair, the method has drawbacks. It is dependent on the skill of the ultrasonographer, and is difficult in obese patients and when a large amount of bowel gas is present. It does, however, have the advantage of allowing studies to be performed at the bedside without the use of contrast agent.

PLAIN X-RAY
We have previously reported the importance of plain abdominal radiographs in monitoring the position of radiopaque parts of the endograft.[20] Movement of the graft attachment device may precede the detection of an endoleak by CT. These findings are significant because they may enable a secondary endoluminal repair to be undertaken before more extensive migration precludes this method of treatment.

MANAGEMENT OF THE ENDOLEAK
Endoleak may be managed by (1) observation; (2) a further endovascular procedure comprising either a supplementary endoluminal repair or embolization; (3) surgical band ligature of the aneurysm neck; and (4) conversion to open repair of the aneurysm.

OBSERVATION
Because a proportion of endoleaks will seal spontaneously, the majority of vascular surgeons are prepared to observe endoleaks, despite the knowledge that aneurysm rupture may occur in patients with this clinical course. Although there is no proof that spontaneous sealing of an endoleak by thrombosis removes systemic arterial pressure from the aneurysm sac, there is presumptive evidence that this is so in the form of reduction in the diameter of aneurysms in

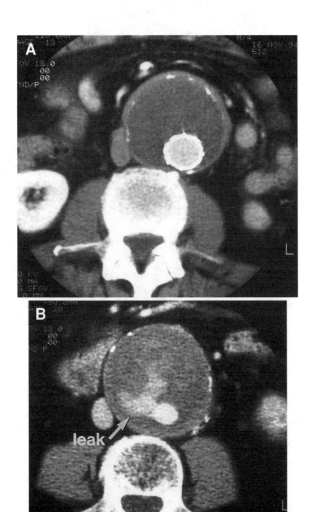

FIGURE 4.

A, contrast CT scan demonstrating exclusion of the aneurysm sac from the circulation. **B,** typical CT appearance of endoleak. Contrast is seen outside the walls of the endovascular graft *(arrow)*. (Reproduced with permission from *Eur J Vasc Endovasc Surg*).

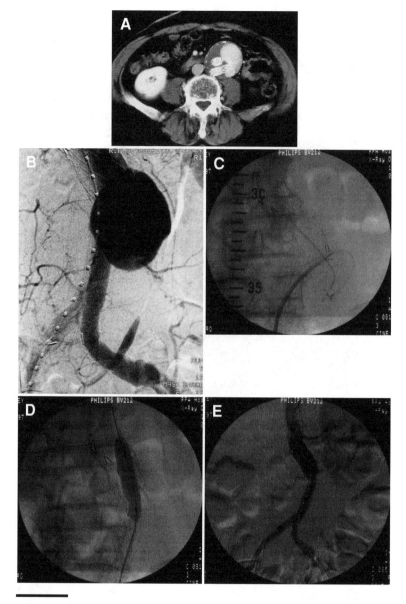

FIGURE 5.

A, contrast CT 1 year after previously successful bifurcated endovascular graft. Note endoleak arising from the contralateral stump on the *left* and the previously vertical contralateral limb lying horizontally. **B,** on-table preprocedure angiogram performed during secondary endoluminal repair. Note the endoleak and complete dislocation of the contralateral limb (<)

Continued

this situation. The duration of observation varies according to the size of the aneurysm. Patient safety would dictate that aneurysms with a diameter of more than 6 cm should not be observed longer than 3 months. In addition, spontaneous seal is no guarantee that this state will continue indefinitely. It has been our experience that recurrent endoleak may follow spontaneous seal.

FURTHER ENDOVASCULAR PROCEDURES

Type 1 endoleaks may be treated by secondary endoluminal repair using a cuff endograft for a proximal endoleak, an extension endograft for a distal iliac endoleak, and an inter-segmental endograft for distraction of component parts of a modular graft (Fig 5). A distal endoleak from a tube endograft may be treated either by (1) a cuff endograft; or (2) conversion to an endoluminal aortoiliac graft with crossover graft and interruption of the contralateral common iliac artery; or (3) conversion to an endoluminal bifurcated graft. Coil embolization has also been used in the treatment of type 1 endoleaks. The place of this maneuver, in the authors' opinion, remains to be established.

Type 2 endoleaks arising from the lumbar arteries may be treated by coil embolization using selective catheterization of branches of the superior gluteal artery (Fig 6). Type 2 endoleaks resulting from retrograde flow in the inferior mesenteric artery have also been treated by embolization using selective catheterization of the middle colic artery.[21]

SURGICAL BAND LIGATURE OF THE AORTIC ANEURYSM NECK

This technique has been reported by the Nottingham group,[22] and involves open exposure and placement of an external ligature to achieve a seal around the proximal graft attachment device. Although requiring laparotomy, it is clearly less disturbing hemodynamically than conversion to open repair in high-risk patients.

FIGURE 5 (cont.)

from the contralateral stump (||). **C,** hard copy from image intensifier demonstrating the capture of a guidewire, passed via a guiding catheter from the left brachial artery, by a goose neck snare passed superiorly through the contralateral limb from the left groin. **D,** traction has been applied to the through and through brachiofemoral guidewire to align the contralateral stump and limb. These have been joined by deployment of a self-expanding intersegmental endograft. **E,** on-table post-procedure angiogram confirming exclusion of the aneurysm sac from the general circulation.

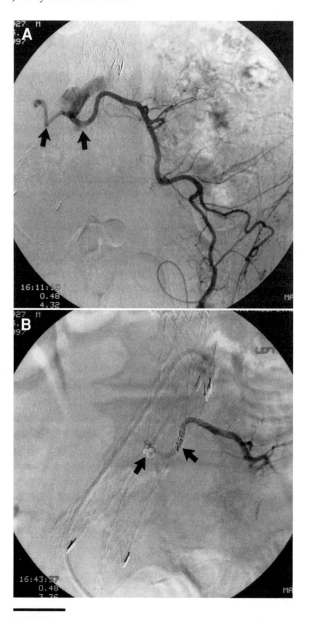

FIGURE 6.

A, selective angiogram demonstrating a type II endoleak arising from the lumbar arteries *(arrows).* The left lumbar artery has been cannulated from the superior gluteal artery via collateral channels. **B,** selective angiogram following coil embolization of the lumbar arteries. Note that bilateral embolization *(arrows)* was required to seal the endoleak and exclude the aneurysm sac from the circulation.

TABLE 2.
Endoleaks: Royal Prince Alfred Hospital, May 1992 Through December 1997 (5½ Years)

Incidence	Operations	200	
	Endoleaks	37 (18.5%)	
Classification	Type 1	28	
	Type 2	9	
Outcome			
	Type 1 (n = 28)		
	Spontaneous seal (1 recurrence)		3
	Successful supplementary endoluminal repair		8
	Conversion (including 3 failed secondary endoluminal repairs)		7
	Surgical ligature of aneurysm neck		1
	No treatment/death and terminal unrelated illness		2
	Observation		7
	Type 2 (n = 9)		
	Spontaneous seal (1 recurrence)		2
	Successful embolization		3
	Observation		4
Summary			
	Sealed (spontaneous and intervention)		16
	Conversion to open		7
	No treatment/death		3
	Persistent endoleak under observation		11

CONVERSION TO OPEN REPAIR

Conversion to open repair may be indicated in situations where supplementary endoluminal repair is not possible or has failed.

MANAGEMENT OF ENDOLEAK AT ROYAL PRINCE ALFRED HOSPITAL, 1992–1997

Endoleak was detected in 37 of 200 endoluminal AAA repair operations (18.5%). Twenty-eight of these were type 1 and 9 were type 2. The outcome in these 37 patients with endoleak is summarized in Table 2. Spontaneous seal occurred in 14%, but recurrent endoleak in 2 patients reduced this to 8%. Significantly, just less than one third of all endoleaks were able to be corrected by a supplementary endovascular procedure. This had the effect of raising the predicted success rate for endoluminal repair at 5 years from 57% to 74% when analyzed by the life table method.

SUMMARY

Endoleak is a unique phenomenon associated with endoluminal deployment of vascular grafts and represents the major challenge with this new technology. The incidence of endoleak may be reduced by improved patient selection and sizing of endografts, combined with good procedural technique. We believe that persistent endoleak is best managed by supplementary endovascular intervention.

REFERENCES

1. May J, White GH, Yu W, et al: Concurrent comparison of endoluminal versus open repair in the treatment of abdominal aortic aneurysms: Analysis of 303 patients by life table method. *J Vasc Surg,* 27:213–222, 1998.
2. White GH, Yu W, May J: "Endoleak": A proposed new terminology to describe incomplete aneurysm exclusion by an endoluminal graft (letter). *J Endovasc Surg* 3:124–125, 1996.
3. White GH, Yu W, May J, et al: Endoleak as a complication of endoluminal grafting of abdominal aortic aneurysms: Classification, incidence, diagnosis, and management. *J Endovasc Surg* 4:152–168, 1997.
4. White GH, May J, Waugh RC, et al: Type I and Type II endoleak: A more useful classification for reporting results of endoluminal repair of AAA (letter). *J Endovasc Surg,* in press.
5. Moore WS, Rutherford R: Transfemoral endovascular repair of abdominal aortic aneurysm: Results of the North American EVT phase 1 trial. *J Vasc Surg* 23:543–553, 1996.
6. Marin ML, Veith F, Cynamon J, et al: Initial experience with transluminally placed endovascular grafts for the treatment of complex vascular lesions. *Ann Surg* 222:449–465, 1995.
7. Blum U, Langer M, Spillner G, et al: Abdominal aortic aneurysms: Preliminary technical and clinical results with transfemoral placement of endovascular self-expanding stent-grafts. *Radiology* 198:25–31, 1996.
8. Parodi JC: Endovascular repair of abdominal aortic aneurysms and other arterial lesions. *J Vasc Surg* 21:549–557, 1995.
9. May J, White GH, Yu W, et al: Surgical management of complications following endoluminal grafting of abdominal aortic aneurysms. *Eur J Vasc Endovasc Surg* 10:51–59, 1995.
10. May J, White G, Yu W, et al: A prospective study of anatomico-pathological changes in abdominal aortic aneurysms following endoluminal repair: Is the aneurysmal process reversed? *Eur J Vasc Endovasc Surg* 12:11–17, 1996.

11. Balm R, Kaatee R, Blankensteijn JD, et al: CT-angiography of abdominal aortic aneurysms after transfemoral endovascular aneurysm management. *Eur J Vasc Endovasc Surg* 12:182–188, 1996.
12. Matsumura JS, Pearce WH, McCarthy WJ, et al: Reduction in aortic aneurysm size: Early results after endovascular graft placement. *J Vasc Surg* 25:113–123, 1997.
13. Bernhard V: Unpublished manuscript presented at International Endovascular Symposium, (1 ES 97), Sydney, Australia, December, 1997.
14. Darling RC, Chang BB, Shah DM, et al: Fate of the excluded abdominal aortic aneurysm sac: Long term follow up of 831 patients. *J Vasc Surg* 24:851–855, 1996.
15. White GH, Yu W, May J, et al: Three-year experience with the White-Yu endovascular GAD graft for transluminal repair of aortic and iliac aneurysms. *J Endovasc Surg* 4:124–136, 1997.
16. Lumsden AB, Allen RC, Chaikof EL, et al: Delayed rupture of aortic aneurysms following endovascular stent grafting. *Am J Surg* 170:174–178, 1995.
17. Stelter W: Unpublished manuscript presented at International Endovascular Symposium (1ES97), Sydney, Australia, December, 1997.
18. Harris PL: Unpublished manuscript presented at International Endovascular Symposium (1ES97), Sydney, Australia, December, 1997.
19. Rozenblit A, Marin ML, Veith F, et al: Endovascular repair of abdominal aortic aneurysm: Value of postoperative follow-up with helical CT: *AJR* 165:1473–1479, 1995.
20. May J, White GH, Waugh R, et al: Importance of plain x-ray in endoluminal aortic graft surveillance. *Eur J Vasc Endovasc Surg* 13:202–206, 1997.
21. Van Schie G, Sieunarine K, Holt M, et al: Successful embolization of persistent endoleak from a patent inferior mesenteric artery. *J Endovasc Surg* 4:312–315, 1997.
22. Yusuf SW, Whitaker SC, Wenham PW, et al: Early results of endovascular abdominal aortic aneurysm repair. *J Endovasc Surg* 3:98A–99A, 1996.

PART III

Venous Disease

CHAPTER 6

Evolution of Varicose Vein Surgery

John J. Bergan, M.D., F.A.C.S., F.R.C.S. (Hon.), Eng.

Professor of Surgery, University of California, San Diego; Professor of Surgery, Loma Linda University Medical Center, Loma Linda, California; Clinical Professor of Surgery, Uniformed Services University of the Health Sciences, Bethesda, Maryland; Professor of Surgery Emeritus, Northwestern University Medical School, Chicago, Illinois

> "Those who do not know history are condemned to relive it."
>
> Santayana

Despite the common occurrence of varicose veins, there are many misconceptions about their etiology, risks, progression, and natural history. Also, there are numerous controversial aspects about evaluation, preoperative diagnosis, and surgery for this condition. Because varicose veins are so common, these differences of opinion assume great importance in patient care. With regard to numbers of patients, it is generally thought that the prevalence of varicose veins in the United States is approximately 10%, but the incidence of this abnormality can be from 10% to 50% depending on the definition used to characterize the condition.

There is still no universal agreement about whether the saphenous vein should be removed or simply ligated when varicose vein surgery is performed. Not long ago complete removal from ankle to groin was routinely done, and this is still the practice of some physicians today. However, reports that the saphenous nerve was injured in ankle-to-groin stripping in up to 10% of cases, as well as pleas from cardiac and arterial surgeons to preserve the saphenous vein for future use as a bypass, convinced many physicians that the saphenous vein should not be removed but instead simply ligated and divided at its junction with the femoral vein.

Widespread use of duplex ultrasonography quickly revealed that the saphenous vein after proximal ligation remained patent, continued to reflux, filled calf varicosities, and was associated with about two thirds of recurrent varicose veins. Because preservation of the saphenous vein remains a desirable goal for some, surgical procedures have been devised to restore competency of the proximal subterminal valve by external banding, or to divert saphenous reflux into the deep venous system by using the principles of conservative hemodynamic treatment of incompetent and varicose veins in ambulatory patients (CHIVA) surgery.

This chapter is based on the following premises: (1) much wisdom can be derived from the experiences of the past; (2) funding is unlikely to become available to support trials that will yield type I evidence on which to base future practice; and (3) treatment of symptoms of venous insufficiency (varicose veins) is important, can yield excellent results, and is extremely satisfying for the patient and surgeon alike.

LESSONS LEARNED FROM THE ANCIENTS

Some of the Greco-Roman era opinions are handed down to us from Hippocrates who recognized venous sclerosis after seeing infection after phlebotomy, from Galen who is credited by some as inventing the ligature, and from Celsus who exposed varicosities through incisions four fingerbreadths apart and cauterized the vein through each incision[1] (Table 1). Celsus then extracted as much of the varix as he could, the principles of midthigh venous interruption and

---

TABLE 1.
Historical Development of Varicose Vein Surgery*

370 BC	Hippocrates	Multiple punctures
50 AD	Celsus	Cautery and/or excision
200	Galen	Hook avulsion
650	Aegineta	Saphenous division, bandaging
1050	Albucasis	Venous stripping (intraluminal)
1550	Paré	Ligation, division
1700	Heister	Bleeding, starvation
1833	Davat	Transcutaneous puncture
1844	Madelung	Saphenous stripping, ligation
1877	Schede	Transcutaneous ligature
1890	Trendelenburg	Saphenous division

*Several early dates are approximate.

stab avulsion of varices were established nearly 2,000 years ago. Some surgeons even today follow these principles.

From the Greco-Roman era to the Renaissance, little surgical knowledge is left to us because of the vast destruction of records that accompanied the successive invasions of Europe by barbaric hordes. A few names descend however. Among these is Guy de Chauliac who opened varices, cauterized the venous ends, and advocated avulsion if the less-invasive method failed. Another is Albucasis who attempted elevation of surgical standards by saying that the practice "had passed into the hands of uncultivated minds." He described multiple vein ligation and external stripping, thus preceding the contribution by Charles Mayo by 900 years.

With regard to venous surgery, the 16th century was marked by the reintroduction of the ligature by Paré, who also recognized the need for pressure and nonelastic support in the healing of venous ulcers.

The most notable contribution of the 17th century was Harvey's description of the circulation of the blood, which in turn was derived from the observations of Fabricius who described the venous valves with remarkable accuracy. However, from a more practical view from the 20th century, Richard Wiseman pointed the way toward successful therapy of severe venous insufficiency. He advocated ". . . a laced-up stocking." For this he used soft dog skin leather,[2] thus uncovering the fact that in treatment of the most severe forms of venous insufficiency, a nonelastic support must be used.

It was John Hunter whose observations dominate the history of diagnosis and treatment of venous disorders in the 18th century. However, he was more concerned with thrombophlebitis than surgical treatment, and correctly separated septic from spontaneous venous thrombosis. As the century turned, the dominant figure whom we observe is Sir Benjamin Brodie. He described saphenous reflux and the test that came to be credited almost 100 years later to Trendelenburg. Although he advocated surgery, the problem of sepsis discouraged him and he later advocated a system of double bandaging in the treatment of venous ulcers. He was extremely successful surgically and financially, so by the time he was knighted by Queen Victoria he was quoted as saying, "Gentleman, there is more in the veins than just blue blood."[1]

It would be improper to leave the 19th century without mentioning Friedrich Trendelenburg. Although a number of surgical procedures including pulmonary embolectomy carry his name, his contribution in varicose vein surgery was saphenous ligation. His incision was at the junction of the middle and upper third of the thigh, and could not have included a proper groin incision. These two errors have been carried down to the present day.

THE 20TH CENTURY

Just after the turn of the century, a simultaneous generation of ideas occurred (Table 2). William Keller invented inversion stripping of the saphenous vein with an intraluminal wire in 1905, Charles Mayo developed the external ring stripper in 1906, and Stephen Babcock advocated an intraluminal rod in 1907. Thus the modern operation is nearly 100 years old and, in Europe, is still referred to as Babcock's operation.

Although venous surgery was a chief concern of vascular surgery during the first half of the 20th century, little was added that was lasting. One negative contribution is worth mentioning; that is, the addition of infusion of sclerotherapeutic agents into the saphenous vein after proximal ligation and division. This was a common part of surgical practice even after World War II but was abandoned after massive recanalization of the saphenous vein was observed. Also, radiologic evidence established that the agents introduced into the superficial system found their way into the deep veins. That ultrasound-guided sclerotherapy of the saphenous

---

TABLE 2.
20th Century Development of Varicose Vein Surgery

1904	Tavel	Saphenous division, injection
1905	Keller	Intraluminal stripping
1906	Mayo	Extraluminal stripping
1907	Babcock	Intraluminal stripping
1908	Schiassi	Sclerotherapy and surgery
1916	Homans	Saphenous ligation
1930	deTakats	Outpatient surgery
1946	—	Demise of operative sclerotherapy
1970	Folse	Doppler reflux detection
1980	—	Duplex venous testing
1989	Strandness/Nicolaides	Quantitative duplex testing
1990	Numerous	Comparative studies

vein is being reintroduced is a tribute to the wisdom of Santayna quoted above.

PATHOPHYSIOLOGY

To understand the modern surgical approach for varicose veins, it is necessary to understand the pathophysiologic state that is being corrected. Initial attempts to unravel the pathophysiology included venous pressure studies, which proved too global in the limb rather than venous-segment specific, and are objectionable to the patient as well. However, these studies have shown that there are two distinct sources of venous hypertension that should be corrected surgically. The first is gravitational and is a result of venous blood coursing in a distal direction down linear axial venous segments, the saphenous veins. This is referred to as hydrostatic pressure and is the weight of the blood column from the right atrium. The highest pressure generated by this mechanism is evident at the ankle and foot where measurements are expressed in centimeters of water or millimeters of mercury.[3] While it is logical to interrupt this pressure column by proximal saphenous ligation, venous anatomy and failure of protective check valves defeat this maneuver.

The second source of venous hypertension is dynamic. This is the force of muscular contraction, usually contained within the compartments of the lower extremity. This high pressure is transmitted through failed perforating veins that penetrate the deep crural fascia.[4] Although many of these perforating veins have no valves, their anatomical angulation prevents reflux into the subcutaneous tissues under normal conditions. Normal valves, present in some of the perforating veins, allow blood flow to be directed from the superficial to the deep tissues. The anatomical angulation and competent valves may be referred to as check mechanisms that protect the venules of the subcutaneous tissue and skin from compartmental hypertension. Failure of this mechanism allows intercompartmental forces to be transmitted directly to unsupported subcutaneous veins and dermal capillaries. These pressures are expressed in hundreds of millimeters of mercury rather than millimeters of water.

Both of the hydraulic forces act on tributaries to the saphenous veins, the reticular veins, and even skin postcapillary venules. It is these pressures acting on a predisposed genetic/hormonal substrate that cause elongation and dilation of the affected vessels. Although the mechanisms and effects are the same, these abnormalities are arbitrarily differentiated into telangiectasias, reticular varicosities, and varicose veins.

SURGICAL OBJECTIVES

An understanding of the source of venous hypertension and its differentiation into hydrostatic and hydrodynamic components is important. The presence of hydrostatic reflux requires surgical correction of this abnormality by disconnecting (and removing) the axial conduits. The presence of hydrodynamic reflux requires ablation of the perforating vein mechanism that exposes the subcutaneous circulation to compartmental pressures. Although this can be achieved by selective perforating vein interruption, it is best done for varicose veins by stab avulsion.

When surgery is decided upon, the goals are to permanently remove the varicosities with the sources of venous hypertension in as cosmetic a fashion as possible with a minimum number of complications. The sources of venous hypertension are described above. Removal of gravitational reflux by axial vein removal and detachment of hydrodynamic forces by superficial varicosity excision accomplish both objectives. Experience in treating recurrent varicose veins has revealed that an inadequate procedure at the saphenofemoral junction is a principal finding. An equally important cause of recurrent varicosities is failure of the primary surgery to completely remove the existing varicosities.

SURGICAL TECHNIQUE

The planned operation for a given patient must be completely individualized. Doppler and duplex studies have shown that in 70% of limbs selected for surgery, typical saphenofemoral reflux will be present. In these, the saphenous vein at the femoral junction must be operated on. However, atypical varicosities without saphenofemoral junction reflux do occur in some 20% of limbs. Others have atypical reflux points causing their varicosities.[5] Clearly, no standard operation fits every patient perfectly.

LIGATION VERSUS STRIPPING

Retrospective reviews of surgical experience are looked upon with disfavor today. Yet a thread of wisdom can be found in some such studies. References to these studies can be found in reference 8. Lofgren et al. examined limbs of patients up to 5 years after high saphenous ligation after stripping compared to 40% after high tie.[6]

This and other studies were dismissed by Dormandy in their prospective, randomized study. They compared saphenous vein stripping and stab avulsion with saphenous high tie and midthigh perforator interruption, finding no differences in either patient or physician evaluation at 3 years.[7] Results of this study were criticized because evaluation was entirely subjective rather than objective. Yet the observations favored stripping.

Now there have been six prospective studies in addition to the study by Dormandy comparing stripping of the saphenous vein with high ligation.[8] The Middlesex group, in their prospective, randomized study, used duplex scanning for postoperative examination of valvular incompetence and photoplethysmography (PPG) as a measure of overall venous function. "Both objective tests of venous function and subjective assessment suggest that the results 21 months after surgery . . . are improved by . . . long saphenous vein stripping from groin to calf." At Maastrict, stripping and ligation were prospectively randomized. Physician and patient assessment of results at 3 years was supplemented by Doppler ultrasound examination with the conclusion that ". . . the results remained significantly better for the stripping group . . ."

In Copenhagen, Jakobsen's prospective evaluation (confirmed by Carl Arnoldi) concluded that saphenous varices are best treated by radical operation (stripping as compared with high tie) in spite of the significantly longer period of disability. In the New Zealand trial, each patient served as his own control, and evaluation was by a single observer at intervals up to 3–5 years after operation. Results, judged only by incidence of varicosities, ". . . were significantly better in limbs from which the long saphenous vein had been stripped. However, saphenous nerve paresthesias biased patient evaluation against ankle-to-groin stripping." At Lund, conventional subjective and objective evaluation was supplemented by foot volumetry before and after treatment. The authors concluded that "this study clearly supports the conclusion that CST (compression sclerotherapy) alone or in combination with high tie cannot replace radical surgery (saphenous stripping, perforator interruption, and stab avulsion) for varicose vein disease with saphenous incompetence."

Only Hammarstein's study concluded ". . . that the removal of the saphenous vein per se is of no therapeutic value if all perforators have been ligated." However, as he emphasized in a later letter, only "by means of a thorough (ascending and descending) phlebographic mapping of the insufficient perforators . . . was precise perforator ligation possible." In commenting on this, Darke suggested that with regard to elimination of perforator-induced saphenous recurrence, ". . . the simplest and least costly and uncomplicated way of eradicating the problem is to remove the saphenous trunk along with the existing and potentially incompetent perforators."

The fate of the long saphenous vein after proximal ligation has been defined by duplex scanning. The evaluation by Rutherford et al. showed that only 8–10 cm of proximal saphenous vein was obliterated after high ligation. They found that all saphenous veins were patent postligation.[9] Friedell studied patients in Florida at a mean follow-up of 10 months and found 78% of saphenous veins completely patent, 15% with less than 10 cm obliterated, and only 7% with a greater length obliterated. In Cardiff, 75 limbs were assessed at a mean follow-up of 1 year by duplex scans. In 49 limbs (65%) the entire saphenous vein was patent from ankle to groin. In 2 additional limbs, less than 5 cm was lost proximally. In a physiologic evaluation of high saphenous ligation using duplex scans and PPG, the Middlesex group found persistent reflux in 24 of 52 limbs with successful proximal ligation. The authors concluded that "a satisfactory outcome was associated with absence of reflux down the long saphenous vein after operation . . . and this operation fails to control functionally significant reflux within the long saphenous vein in a high proportion of cases."[10]

The techniques of saphenous surgery are well described in standard surgical texts, but it is their outpatient variations that have come into vogue. Removal of a saphenous vein is now done by groin-to-knee downward stripping of the varicose veins.[11] Techniques to decrease hematomas after downward stripping include adrenalin gauze packing of the saphenectomy tunnel. Tourniquet use during saphenous stripping is very important in surgery of massive varices and those of the Klippel-Trenaunay syndrome.

A short (2 cm) inguinal crease incision and superficial fascia division exposes saphenous tributaries. These are drawn into the incision beyond primary and even secondary tributaries, which are electrocoagulated. The large medial posterior tributary (termination of Giacomini vein) is controlled, and saphenous duplication is searched for. The saphenous vein is divided, its termination suture-ligated, and the intraluminal stripper passed distally. It is identified and brought externally through a 2- to 3-mm stab incision in the region of the knee.

Large proximal tributaries may represent a form of saphenous duplication. These are cannulated to determine their courses and excised. With the leg extended and the thigh and leg elevated 30 degrees, the vein is inverted into itself over the Codman plastic stripper without any attached head. A heavy suture is ligated to attach the vein to the stripper before the invagination maneuver. A

10-cm gauze strip soaked in 0.5% lidocaine with epinephrine 1:100,000 is tied to the stripper at the point of vein ligation. This will be drawn into the saphenous vein as it is inverted. Traction will be delivered from the plastic stripper to the gauze pack, and the vein will not be torn.

Stripping of the saphenous vein should be delayed until the operation of stab avulsion of varices is completed. The stripping produces proximal venous spasm and distal venous hypertension. This in turn increases blood loss during stab avulsion.

Stab avulsion is practiced using vertical incisions except at the groin, knee, and ankle where they should conform to transverse skin lines. Incisions are limited to 2–3 mm in length and an attempt is made to separate them more than 10–12 cm from one another. All previously marked varicose clusters are removed. Success of surgery is directly related to completeness of removal of these varices in as cosmetic a manner as is possible. There is no need to dissect out individual perforating veins nor to ligate them either above or below the fascia. The entire cannulated saphenous vein is removed distally, and the gauze pack is left in place while stab avulsion incisions are sutured. Each incision is closed with fine interrupted, inverted intradermal suture, and the closure is reinforced with paper tape. It is recognized that suture closure of these small incisions may be unnecessary.

RESULTS OF VARICOSE VEIN SURGERY

In a recent 24-month period, 281 limbs of 238 patients (36 men) were operated on for primary venous insufficiency. All operations were performed on an outpatient basis. Only three patients required hospitalization, one for seizures and two for significant pain.

The most common postoperative complication was ecchymosis in the medial thigh in its proximal third. While none of this ecchymosis required treatment, in two patients hyperpigmentation occurred either in that area or distally in the calf. Ecchymosis was occasionally seen in the retromalleolar area, indicating that bleeding had occurred beneath the deep fascia of the leg. The next most frequent complication, the appearance of lymphoceles, was unexpected and occurred in five cases. These were usually along the path of stripping of the greater saphenous vein, either in the thigh or in tributaries to the saphenous vein in the leg. None of the lymphoceles required treatment and all resolved spontaneously. There were two wound infections, both in the groin. Neither required surgical debridement or surgical closure, and both healed with antibiotic coverage. Transient numbness in the saphenous nerve distribution was present in 19 cases. This was invariably traced to a site of stab avulsion.

One unusual complication, a posterior tibial nerve injury at the ankle, caused significant disability and required physical therapy. This resolved after 7 months and was caused by surgery on a retromalleolar perforating vein to diminish the effects of a corona phlebectatica.

Reoperations within this 2-year period were required in four cases. All involved the greater saphenous vein, which had been ligated in two and stripped in two. Upon review of the operative notes in the latter two cases, it is apparent that a missed duplicated or parallel tributary vein was the cause for the need for reoperation.

It should be noted that in the two cases of deliberate ligation of the saphenous vein rather than stripping, a radical operation was done removing the proximal 10–15 cm of the greater saphenous vein and avulsion of tributaries beyond their primary or secondary branchings. Therefore, the recurrence was from communicating veins or perforating veins distal to the ligation site. This emphasizes the need for short stripping of the saphenous vein rather than high ligation.

CONCLUSION

Although this description of the evolution of varicose vein surgery from its beginnings to the end of the 20th century will not convince every physician or surgeon that varicose veins should be operated upon or how this should be done, it does provide a summary of a single point of view. This is summarized in the statement that the best treatment given is that which is best available to the patient at the time therapy is decided upon and accomplished.

REFERENCES

1. Rose SS: Historical development of varicose vein surgery, in Bergan JJ, Goldman MP (eds): *Varicose Veins and Telangiectasias: Diagnosis and Treatment*. St. Louis, Quality Medical Publishing, 1993.
2. Bergan JJ: Historical highlights in treating venous insufficiency, in Bergan JJ, Yao JST (eds): *Venous Disorders*. Philadelphia, WB Saunders, 1991.
3. Bjordal RI: Pressure and flow measurements in venous insufficiency of the legs, in Eklof B, Gjöres JE, Thulesius O, et al (eds): *Controver-*

sies in the Management of Venous Disorders. London, Butterworth, 1989.

4. Arnoldi CC: Venous pressure in patients with valvular incompetence of the veins of the lower extremities. *Acta Chir Scand* 132:628–645, 1966.

5. Goren G, Yellin AE: Primary varicose veins: Topographic and hemodynamic considerations. *J Cardiovasc Surg* 31:672–677, 1990.

6. Lofgren KA, Ribisi AP, Myers TT: An evaluation of stripping versus ligation for varicose veins. *Arch Surg* 76:310–316, 1958.

7. Woodyer AB, Reddy PJ, Dormandy JA: *Should We Strip the Long Saphenous Vein?* London, John Libbey, 1986, pp 151–154.

8. Bergan JJ: Saphenous stripping and quality of outcome. *Br J Surg* 83:1025–1027, 1996.

9. Rutherford RB, Sawyer JD, Jones DN: The fate of residual saphenous vein after partial removal or ligation. *J Vasc Surg* 12:422–428, 1990.

10. McMullin GM, Coleride Smith PD, Scurr JH: Objective assessment of high ligation without stripping the long saphenous vein. *Br J Surg* 78:1139–1142, 1991.

11. Bergan JJ. Surgical management of primary and recurrent varicose veins, in Gloviczki P, Yao JST (eds): *Handbook of Venous Disorders.* London, Chapman & Hall, 1996.

CHAPTER 7

Balloon Dissection for Endoscopic Subfascial Ligation

Roy L Tawes, M.D.
Chief of Surgery, Mills Peninsula Hospital, Burlingame, California;
Clinical Professor of Surgery, University of California at San Francisco,
San Francisco, California

L. Albert Wetter, M.D.
Mills Peninsula Hospital, Burlingame, California; Instructor in Surgery,
University of California at San Francisco, San Francisco, California

Gerald R. Sydorak, M.D.
Clinical Associate Professor of Surgery, University of California at San
Francisco, San Francisco, California; Staff Vascular Surgeon, Mills
Peninsula Hospital, Burlingame, California

George D. Hermann, B.S.M.E.
General Manager, Fogarty Research, Portola Valley, California

Thomas J. Fogarty, M.D.
Professor of Surgery, Stanford University Medical Center, Stanford,
California

C hronic venous insufficiency of the lower extremities is a debilitating disease affecting more than 2.5 million Americans.[1] Linton[2] and Cockett and Jones[3] have identified perforating vein incompetence as an important contributing factor. The traditional surgical solution of directly exposing these vessels via a long overlying incision was fraught with a high rate of wound healing complications.[4, 5]

The proliferation of laparoscopic instrumentation and techniques, as well as the availability of duplex ultrasound imaging, has created an opportunity to improve the surgical treatment of this disease. The endoscopic approach to perforating vein ligation was pioneered by Hauer in 1986.[6] This approach is often referred to as

Advances in Vascular Surgery®, vol. 6
© 1998, Mosby, Inc.

subfascial endoscopic perforator surgery (SEPS). Since Hauer's initial work, the endoscopic approach has evolved with some specialized instrumentation and techniques,[7] including the use of balloon dissection.[8]

PATIENT EVALUATION AND SELECTION

Patients with advanced stasis dermatatis with or without active ulceration are sent to the noninvasive vascular laboratory for documentation of venous incompetence by duplex ultrasound. The disease states of these patients correspond to classes C4, C5, and C6 according to the CEAP (Clinical status, Etiology, Anatomy, Pathophysiology) classification system for venous disease.[9] The superficial, perforator, and deep venous systems are evaluated. For the SEPS procedure to be performed, the deep system must be patent and there must be documentation of reflux of the perforator system. If superficial incompetence is identified as well, saphenous stripping may also be performed at the time of surgery. Documented recent deep venous thrombosis is not necessarily a contraindication provided recanalization has occurred.

Duplex scanning performed on the day of surgery is helpful for marking the specific location of the incompetent perforators. The location of the saphenous vein is marked so that it can be avoided during trocar placement. It should be noted that duplex scanning will not yield a false-positive result. However, duplex may not identify all incompetent perforators. Consequently, we routinely interrupt all perforators we encounter at the time of surgery.

INSTRUMENTATION

Most of the equipment needed to perform these procedures is the same as that needed to perform laparoscopic cholecystectomy. This includes the laparoscopic cart (video camera and monitor, light source, carbon dioxide insufflator), a 10-mm laparoscope (0 or 30 degree), and 5-mm endoscopic instruments (cannula, grasper, shears). No additional capital equipment expenditure is necessary to begin performing the SEPS procedure with the balloon technique.

Several specific instruments not routinely used with laparoscopic cholecystectomy are important (Fig 1). One is the balloon dissector (General Surgical Innovations, Cupertino, Calif). Although dissection of the subfascial space can be accomplished manually, the large unencumbered working space created by the balloon offers greater exposure than other methods, particularly

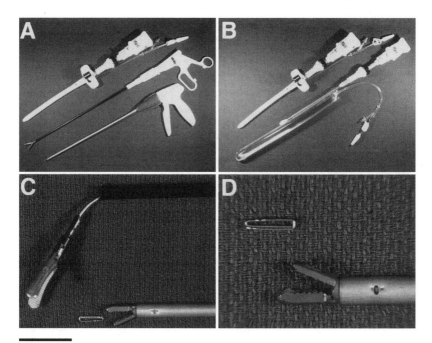

FIGURE 1.

Specialized instrumentation for subfascial endoscopic perforator surgery (SEPS) technique. **A,** balloon dissector *(above)*, 5-mm roticulating grasper, 5-mm clip applier *(below)*. **B,** detail of dissection balloon. Ready for insertion *(above)*, and with cover removed and inflated with 250 mL of saline *(below)*. **C,** tip detail of roticulating grasper that has been articulated *(above)*, and 5-mm clip applier with fired 8-mm clip *(below)*. **D,** clip applier detail shows tri-fold design of 8-mm clip. See color plate 1.

when the dissected space is distended with carbon dioxide. Another item is the 5-mm clip applier (Ethicon Endosurgery, Cincinnati, Ohio). Although 10-mm endoscopic clip appliers have been used successfully in this procedure, the greater visibility and maneuverability offered by the slender 5-mm shaft is very helpful, particularly when working in the more distal subfascial regions. A third instrument is the roticulating endograsper (US Surgical, Norwalk, Conn). The distal shaft of the grasper can articulate 90 degrees, which makes it particularly useful for dissecting along the border of the long tunnel-like subfascial endoscopic working space.

TECHNIQUE

With the patient supine and in Trendelenburg position, the knee is flexed and slightly elevated and the tibia is marked. Anesthesia options include spinal, general, or epidural. We see no need to use a tourniquet. Perforating veins are easier to identify under physiologic pressures.

The primary port is placed a full handsbreadth below the popliteal crease and two fingerbreadths medial to the tibia. The marked perforators should be used as a guide for optimal position of this incision. Using a #15 blade, a 10- to 15-mm incision is made over the medial aspect of the superficial posterior compartment. Initial separation is conducted with a Metzenbaum scissors; thereafter a pair of Army-Navy retractors are used to bluntly dissect the subcutaneous tissue down to the fascia until the shimmering white surface of the fascia is clearly identified. Confirming the nerve is not present, a No. 15 blade is once again used to make a 1-cm incision in the fascia, just enough to expose the muscle without penetrating into it. It is important to keep the fascial incision as close to 1 cm as possible because a larger incision will tend to promote gas leakage around the cannula. A small finger can be used to develop an initial pocket in the subfascial space. An Allis clamp can be used to retract the inferior fascial incision to facilitate insertion of the balloon dissector into the subfascial space. With the dissector's olive tip introduced under the inferior flap of the fascial incision, the balloon dissector is carefully advanced subfascially and directed toward the medial malleolus.

After the balloon is fully inserted, the black lever on the balloon cover is depressed to allow withdrawal of the peel-away cover. Pulling the balloon cover straight back and slightly upwards exposes the balloon inside the subfascial space. It is important to make sure that any exposed balloon is completely advanced within the subfascial space before iniating balloon inflation. The suction outlet is closed and the balloon is inflated with 200–300 mL of normal saline using a pair of 60-mL syringes (Fig 2, A). The balloon is constructed such that it will first expand radially and then distally as the balloon everts. Depending on the length of the patient's leg, full deployment of the dissection balloon may not be necessary to dissect down to the medial malleous. Filling of the balloon can be observed or palpated from outside the leg as the balloon progresses distally to the medial malleolus. External palpation with the hands also enables the surgeon to help direct the balloon's dissection distally.

Once the balloon is adequately inflated, it is then deflated by opening the suction outlet, allowing the balloon to drain. Residual saline is actively aspirated with the syringe or wall suction so as not to enlarge the incison upon balloon removal. When completely

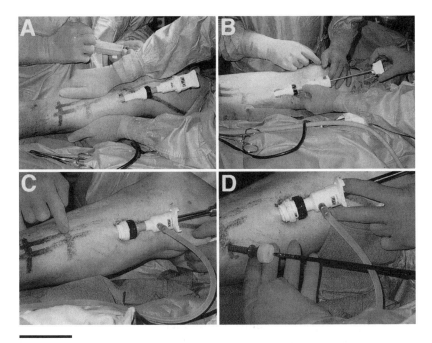

FIGURE 2.

Balloon dissection and port placement. **A,** inflation of dissecting balloon. Surgeon provides external manual compression of proximal calf to facilitate distal propagation of dissection balloon. **B,** removal of obturator, leaving 10-mm cannula in dissected subfascial compartment. **C,** the 10-mm laparoscope is introduced. External finger palpation at duplex marking confirms location of perforator. Note carbon dioxide line is connected to cannula to provide an insufflated subfascial working space. **D,** a grasper is introduced through the secondary 5-mm port. See color plate 2.

evacuated, the balloon is removed by pulling back on the balloon filler tube. After depressing the black buttons on the housing, the guide rod is withdrawn from the cannula (Fig 2, B). The cannula is then rotated into position so that the threads on the cannula seal engage the fascial incision to create an airtight seal. The insufflation line is attached to the cannula, and the dissected space is insufflated with carbon dioxide at 15 mm Hg with medium or high flow. A zero-degree, 10-mm scope is inserted into the dissected space (Fig 2, C).

A large, clean working space typically extending down to the level of the medial malleolus is observed on the video monitor. The camera and scope are rotated to an orientation such that the fascia is seen above and the muscle lies below. Under direct endoscopic visualization with transillumination, the 5-mm secondary trocar is introduced, taking care to avoid any vessels. Proper placement of this port is critical to achieve the best range of motion for instrument manipulation. To get optimal access to the distal perforators and to avoid "sword fighting" with the instruments, the secondary port should be placed at least 2 fingerbreadths posterior and 3 fingerbreadths inferior to the primary port (Fig 2, D).

It is not uncommon to observe freely exposed perforating veins immediately after introduction of the scope. More frequently, however, a modest amount of dissection (usually on the tibial margin of the dissected space) is required to fully expose the perforating vein. The skin markings from the prior duplex examination can be particularly helpful in guiding the surgeon to the appropriate area. External palpation over the markings can be observed endoscopically. Likewise, the bright light from the endoscope can be viewed through the skin to further orient the surgeon and to help identify venous structures. After the perforator is identifed endoscopically and sufficiently exposed with a 5-mm dissecting grasper (Fig 3), the perforator is double clipped with a 5-mm endoscopic clip applier. In general, the perforators are not divided—it takes additional time and venous reflux is sufficiently interrupted with the clips. However, occasionally the clipped perforators can interfere with distal access, in which case they can be promptly divided with endoscopic shears. All perforators that can be identified are interrupted. It is necessary to pay particular attention to the area immediately adjacent to the ulcer so as not to miss perforators contributing to the clinical problem.

Occasionally, at the malleolar level, a duplex marking does not reveal a corresponding perforator endoscopically. In these instances, it is necessary to explore the deep compartment. Anatomically speaking, in the more proximal portion of the calf, the perforating veins communicate between the deep and superficial venous systems by routinely traversing the superficial posterior compartment. However, at the level of the malleolus, the perforators are often seen to traverse the deep posterior compartment instead.[10] Therefore, in these instances, the deep fascia must be dissected and the deep compartment must be explored. Fortunately, the deep fascia is relatively friable and can be taken down endoscopically with little difficulty. In most cases, an elusive malleolar perforator can be found in this region and subsequently clipped. In these cases, use of the balloon dissector is particularly helpful because it facilitates optimal exposure in this area. Figure 4 shows an example of successfully accessing the deep compartment at the malleolar level using this technique. In some cases after balloon deflation,

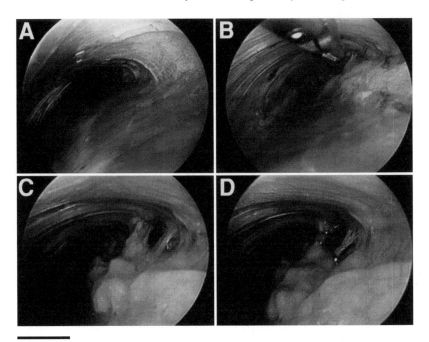

FIGURE 3.

Endoscopic exposure and interruption of perforating vein. **A,** view of insufflated subfascial compartment immediately after balloon dissection. Note fascia above, muscle below, and connective tissue at tibial margin. **B,** dissecting grasper advanced toward perforator on right. **C,** additional dissection with grasper exposed perforator, in preparation for clipping. **D,** perforating vein after clips applied. See color plate 3.

the balloon can be repositioned and reinflated to provide additional working space in the malloeolar region.

In general, it is more difficult to maneuver the scope and instrumentation at the malleolar level than at midcalf. In some instances, it can be useful to insert another 5-mm working port several centimeters inferior to the prior secondary port. This placement improves triangulation of the instruments in the malleolar region yet is still remote from the area of pathologic skin changes.

After interruption of the perforators, the trocars are removed, hemostasis is checked, and the incisions are closed in the usual manner. The fascial defects are not closed. If superficial stripping is indicated, it is performed at this time in the standard manner. All wounds are covered with nonadherent dressings, and the leg is wrapped with 4- and 6-inch Ace bandages from the forefoot to the upper calf or leg as indicated. The patient is observed in the

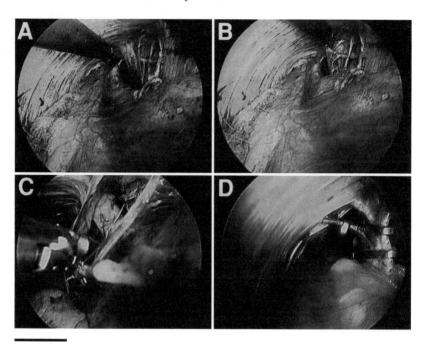

FIGURE 4.
Endoscopic technique of perforator interruption in deep fascial compartment. **A**, view of dissected space. Tip of grasper is at level of malleolus. The deep fascia, which separates the superficial compartment from the deep compartment, is just to the right of the grasper. **B**, grasper easily divides deep fascia. **C**, deep fasica is retracted with grasper to expose a significant perforator at level of malleolus. **D**, view of perforator in deep fascial compartment with clipping complete. See color plate 4.

recovery room for several hours with the legs elevated, and is discharged the same day. The elastic wrap is replaced with compression stockings after 24–48 hours, and the patient is followed up routinely on an outpatient basis after 1 week. Some patients with active ulceration may require Unna's boots for 3–6 weeks postoperatively.

DISCUSSION

We have performed 110 procedures using this technique with balloon dissection and have found the technique to be relatively straightforward, with a routine endoscopic operating time of 20–30 minutes. In many instances, additional ligation and stripping of varicose, greater saphenous, or lesser saphenous veins follows the SEPS procedure. Complications have been minimal, with no compartment syndrome and no bleeding problems. We have been impressed with the high degree of patient satisfaction. During the course of performing these procedures, we have progressively become more aggressive in pursuing this surgical approach. The pain and poor wound healing often associated with lipodermatosclerosis and venous claudication are sufficient clinical indications for this type of procedure. If compression therapy is not showing clinical improvement, it makes little sense to wait for a C4 or C5 patient to deteriorate to a C6 level whereby Unna's boots and other ulcer maintenance steps must be implemented.

Early results have been gratifying. In 110 procedures, all but 10 patients were discharged the same day as surgery (8 were observed overnight and 2 were hospitalized longer for cardiac complications). In 6 patients, healing was not accomplished. Subsequent duplex evaluation revealed a missed perforator at the time of surgery in 4 patients. Two other patients had recurrence of their symptoms 12 and 18 months after SEPS, respectively. Both of these patients underwent redo SEPS without difficulty and were relieved of their symptoms. The expected economic benefits (shortened length of stay, reduced reliance on chronic ulcer maintenance) is significant in the present managed care environment.

Overall, we have found this balloon dissection technique to significantly augment the endoscopic working space for the SEPS procedure. This improved exposure expedites the identification, dissection, and clipping of the perforating veins. There is a very short learning curve after introduction to the proper technique. This particular technique brings the procedure to within the skill level of many surgeons who may not possess appreciable prior endoscopic surgery experience.

REFERENCES

1. Gloviczki P, Cambria RA, Rhee RY, et al: Surgical technique and preliminary results of endoscopic subfascial division of perforating veins. *J Vasc Surg* 23:517–523, 1996.
2. Linton R: The communicating veins of the lower leg and the operative technique for their ligation. *Ann Surg* 107:582–593, 1938.
3. Cockett F, Jones B: The ankle blow-out syndrome: A new approach to the varicose ulcer problem. *Lancet* 1:17–23, 1953.
4. Wilkinson GE, Maclaren IF: Long term review of procedures for venous perforator insufficiency. *Surg Gynecol Obstet* 163:117–120, 1986.
5. Cockett FB: Indications for and complications of the ankle perforator exploration. *Phlebologie* 3:3–6, 1988.
6. Hauer G: The endoscopic subfascial division of the perforating veins: Preliminary report (in German). *VASA* 14:59–61, 1985.

7. Gloviczki P, Bergan JB, Menawat SS, et al: Safety, feasibility and early efficacy of subfascial endoscopic perforator surgery: A preliminary report from the North American registry. *J Vasc Surg* 25:94–105, 1997.

8. Tawes RL, Wetter LA, Hermann GD, et al: Endoscopic technique for subfascial perforating vein interruption. *J Endovasc Surg* 3:414–420, 1996.

9. Executive Committee of the American Venous Forum: Classification and grading disease in the lower limbs: A consensus statement, in Gloviczki P, Yao JT (eds): *Handbook of Venous Disorders.* London, Chapman & Hall Medical, 1996, pp 652–660.

10. Mozes G, Gloviczki P, Menawat SS, et al: Surgical anatomy for endoscopic subfascial division of the perforating veins. *J Vasc Surg* 24:800–808, 1996.

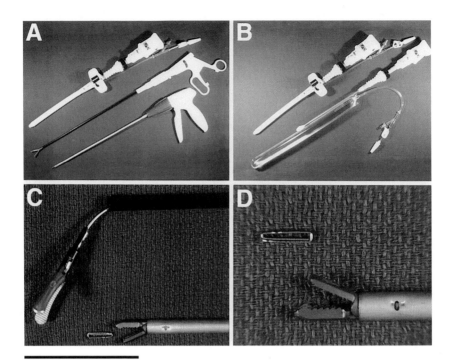

TAWES COLORPLATE 1.

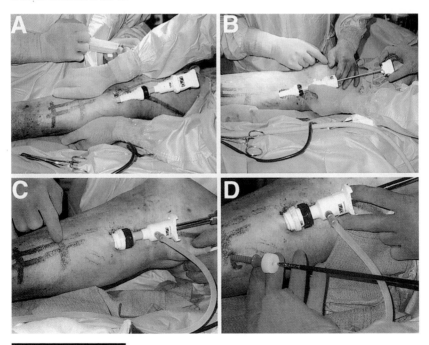

TAWES COLORPLATE 2.

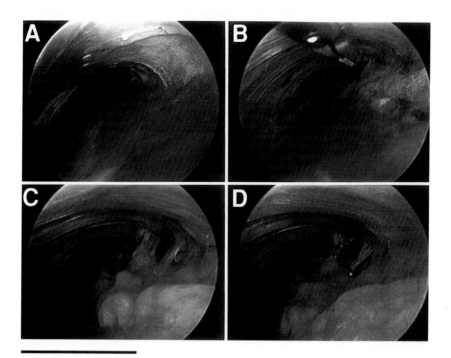

TAWES COLORPLATE 3.

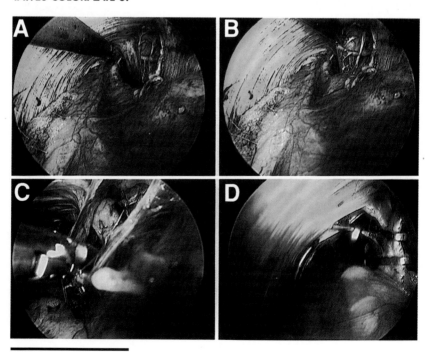

TAWES COLORPLATE 4.

CHAPTER 8

Renal Revascularization for Salvage: Results of Treatment for Renal Artery Occlusion

Kimberley J. Hansen, M.D.
Associate Professor of Surgery, Department of General Surgery, Wake Forest University School of Medicine, Winston-Salem, North Carolina

Timothy C. Oskin, M.D.
Vascular Surgery Fellow, Department of General Surgery, Wake Forest University School of Medicine, Winston-Salem, North Carolina

T raditional management of renovascular disease has focused on renovascular hypertension, yet atherosclerotic renovascular occlusive disease is an anatomically progressive disease that may lead to inadequate renal plasma flow and concomitant decline in excretory renal function. Recent reports have emphasized the potential for retrieval of excretory renal function in select patients with renovascular hypertension and renal dysfunction.[1] These observations have renewed awareness of the functional consequences of renal ischemia and have led to the term *ischemic nephropathy*. By definition ischemic nephropathy reflects the presence of anatomically severe renal occlusive disease in a patient with excretory renal insufficiency. Studies from our center suggest that the decline in renal function associated with ischemic nephropathy may be rapid and consistent with early entry into dialysis-dependent renal failure.[2] Although surgical therapy has improved excretory renal function and decreased the subsequent rate of decline in function on follow-up,[1] results from renal duplex sonography (RDS) in consecutive patients considered for chronic renal replacement therapy suggest that up to 20% of patients reaching dialysis dependence may have ischemic nephropathy.[3] Moreover, among patients with dialysis-dependent ischemic nephropathy,

70% of patients with bilateral renovascular disease or its equivalence have been removed permanently from dialysis dependence after operation.[2] For both azotemic and dialysis-dependent patients, improved excretory renal function is associated with significant improvement in estimated survival.[1, 2] Based on these collective data, a management strategy that optimizes recovery of renal function would appear to provide the best quality and quantity of life. In this regard, our operative management emphasizes complete renal revascularization for hemodynamically significant renovascular disease in preference to nephrectomy.

Renal artery occlusion (RA-OCC) represents the final expression of anatomically progressive atherosclerotic occlusive disease. In a prospective study of the anatomical and functional changes during drug therapy for renovascular hypertension secondary to atherosclerotic renal artery disease, 12% with significant stenosis progressed to total occlusion.[4] When a high-grade stenosis progresses to complete occlusion, RA-OCC may be clinically silent or present with worsening of previously controlled hypertension and elevated serum creatinine levels. In this latter instance, nephrectomy and renal artery revascularization are equally effective in the treatment of hypertension originating from RA-OCC; however, renal artery revascularization has the best opportunity to improve renal function. Moreover, a conservative approach toward nephrectomy is warranted because hemodynamically significant contralateral stenosis develops in more than 35% of patients with atherosclerotic lesions during follow-up.[5] A stenosis in the contralateral kidney after nephrectomy places the patient at risk for recurrent hypertension and dialysis-dependent ischemic nephropathy.

Once RA-OCC is identified in a hypertensive patient with poor renal function, the determinants of renal function retrieval are poorly understood. Past recommendations regarding surgical reconstruction for RA-OCC have focused on absolute renal length, angiographic demonstration of a reconstituted distal renal artery, and the results of kidney biopsy. In contrast to those who would recommend nephrectomy based upon these parameters, we reserve nephrectomy for a surgically unreconstructable renal artery to a nonfunctioning kidney.

DIAGNOSTIC EVALUATION

Continued improvement in sonographic technology has made RDS an accurate screening method in identification of renal artery occlusive disease. In the hands of an experienced sonographer, a technically successful RDS study can be obtained in approximately 95% of cases, with a diagnostic accuracy estimated at 96% when a single renal artery is present.[6] Although RDS is unable to evaluate accessory vessels, a negative RDS study effectively excludes significant renovascular disease when ischemic nephropathy is present because an accessory vessel lesion alone does not account for renal insufficiency. Through this approach to preliminary screening with RDS, the use of arteriography can be limited to patients with renal insufficiency associated with either positive findings on RDS or severe hypertension.

We continue to rely on "cut-film" angiography for renal artery imaging. The use of a single midstream flush aortogram requires no more contrast material than that required for multiple intraarterial digital subtraction studies. In addition, standard arteriography provides information concerning cortical thickness and renal length along with improved clarity for interpretation of intrarenal artery anatomy. The fact that arterography can aggravate preexisting renal dysfunction especially in patients with concomitant diabetes is widely recognized, but we believe the risk is justified in patients with ischemic nephropathy and severe/accelerated hypertension. In these circumstances, the potential benefit derived from identification and correction of functionally significant renovascular occlusive lesions exceeds the risk of arteriography.

Because the lower limits of function retrieval are poorly defined, before nephrectomy for RA-OCC in patients with ischemic nephropathy, excretory renal function should be evaluated in the affected kidney. Isotopic renography is used to determine the relative contribution to renal function on the affected side. In the case of a small kidney without a demonstrable nephrogram or reconstituted distal renal artery and minimal function on renogram, we will revascularize the kidney when a normal distal renal artery is demonstrated at operation. In about 40% of such cases, a normal distal vessel will be found and the kidney successfully revascularized. Nevertheless, if atherosclerosis involves the branch vessels to a nonfunctioning kidney, we will proceed with nephrectomy. In this setting, overall excretory function is not diminished.

OPERATIVE MANAGEMENT

To examine the patient population with RA-OCC and results of our management philosophy, we have reviewed our experience in patients with RA-OCC and compared those with patients managed

TABLE 1.

Demographic Characteristics of Patients With Renal Artery Stenosis
(RAS) and Renal Artery Occlusion *(RA-OCC)*

	RAS (*n* = 302)	*RA-OCC* (*n* = 95)	*P*-value
Mean age (yr)	62.7 ± 12	62.6 ± 9	0.91
Gender			0.15
Female	47%	55%	
Male	53%	45%	
SBP(mm Hg)	197 ± 38	204 ± 31	0.08
DBP(mm Hg)	103 ± 22	106 ± 20	0.26
BP medications	2.5 ± 1.1	3.0 ± 1.1	<0.01
SCr (mg/dL)	2.0 ± 1.4	2.8 ± 2.0	<0.01
EGFR (mL/min/m^2)	41 ± 25	32 ± 18	<0.01
Severe renal dysfunction (SCr > 2.0)	35%	60%	<0.01
Dialysis dependence	5%	12%	0.03
Cardiac disease	42%	51%	0.15
Angina	23%	25%	0.71
MI	30%	39%	0.11
CHF	16%	34%	<0.01
CABG/PTCA	13%	12%	0.73
Cerebrovascular disease	28%	23%	0.34
TIA/CVA	23%	18%	0.34
CEA	15%	9%	0.16

Abbreviations: SBP, systolic blood pressure; *DBP,* diastolic blood pressure; *SCr,* serum creatinine; *EGFR,* estimated glomerular filtration rate; *MI,* myocardial infarction; *CHF,* congestive heart failure; *CABG/PTCA,* coronary artery bypass grafting/percutaneous coronary angioplasty; *TIA/CVA,* transient ischemic attack/cerebrovascular accident; *CEA,* carotid endarterectomy.

for renal artery stenosis (RAS) during the same 10-year period.[7] During this period we operated on 397 patients for atherosclerotic renal artery occlusive disease at our center. Within this group, 117 patients were found to have complete occlusion of at least one renal artery. Omitting 22 patients in which occlusion occured acutely or after renal artery intervention, 95 consecutive patients were treated for 100 chronic atherosclerotic renal artery occlusions. This group included 52 women and 43 men with a mean age of 63 ± 9 years (Table 1). All patients had hypertension (mean blood pressure, 204 ± 31/106 ± 20 mm Hg; mean number of antihypertension medications, 3.0 ± 1.1 drugs). Defined as a serum creatinine

TABLE 2.
Operative Procedures Performed in 95
Patients With Renal Artery Occlusion
(RA-OCC)

	Number
No. of patients (total)	95
No. of kidneys (total)	190
No. of kidneys with RA-OCC	100
Revascularization	75
Bypass	56
Thromboendarterectomy	14
Reimplantation	5
Nephrectomy	25
Combined aortic reconstruction	39
Aneurysmal disease	14
Occlusive disease	25

level of 1.3 mg/dL or greater, 84 patients (88%) had renal dysfunction (mean serum creatinine level, 2.8 ± 2.0 mg/dL). Fifty-nine patients (62%) had severe dysfunction, with a serum creatinine level of 2.0 mg/dL or greater, whereas 11 patients (12%) were dialysis dependent. Organ-specific atherosclerotic damage was present in 95% of 95 patients manifest by renal dysfunction in 88%, cardiac disease in 50%, cerebrovascular disease in 23%, significant aortic disease in 73%, and peripheral vascular disease in 31%.

Evaluation of renal vasculature included conventional cut-film angiography in all patients. Angiography demonstrated distal renal artery reconstitution on delayed films to 56 of 81 kidneys (69%), whereas 54 of 87 kidneys (62%) demonstrated a nephrogram. Neither distal reconstitution nor nephrogram was demonstrated in 20 of 79 kidneys (25%). Preoperative kidney length associated with RA-OCC in 77 patients averaged 8.0 ± 1.5 cm.

Ninety-five patients underwent reconstruction for 100 kidneys with RA-OCC. Seventy-five kidneys in 70 patients were revascularized, and 25 nephrectomies were performed for an unreconstructable renal artery lesion (Table 2). Renal artery reconstruction included aortorenal bypass in 56 instances, thromboendarterectomy in 14 instances, and reimplantation in 5 instances. Hemodynamically significant contralateral renal artery occlusive disease requiring reconstruction was present in 59 of 90 patients (66%) with unilateral RA-OCC.

TABLE 3.

Comparison of Operative Results in Patients With Renal
Artery Occlusion by Treatment Group

	Renal Artery Revascularization (n = 70)	Nephrectomy (n = 25)	*P*-value
Perioperative mortality (%)	2.8	12	0.11
Hypertension response (%)			0.54
Cured	10	14	
Improved	82	73	
No change	8	13	
Renal function response (%)*			0.31
Improved	52	39	
No change/ worsened	48	61	

*Preoperative serum creatinine ≥ 1.3 mg/dL.

There were 5 (5.3%) perioperative deaths among the 95
patients treated for RA-OCC. The perioperative mortality rate of
2.8% in the renal artery revascularization group and 12% in the
nephrectomy group did not differ statistically ($P = 0.11$; Table 3).
A similar perioperative mortality rate of 4.0% was observed in the
RAS group ($P = 0.59$; Table 4). During mean follow-up of 32
months, the survival rate did not differ significantly within the RA-
OCC group whether treated by nephrectomy or renal artery revascularization ($P = 0.47$). Multivariate analysis demonstrated a significant and independent association with increased survival and
dialysis-free survival among patients with improved postoperative
estimated glomerular filtration rate, whereas decreased survival
was associated with preoperative age, serum creatinine level, history of congestive heart failure, and level of systolic blood pressure (Table 5). The product-limit estimate of time to death in the
nephrectomy group is depicted by a *solid line* in Figure 1. During
follow-up there were 24 deaths in the RA-OCC group compared
with 37 in the RAS group ($P > 0.01$), whereas the estimated rate of
survival did not differ ($P = 0.14$). By multivariate analysis preoperative age, creatinine level, history of congestive heart failure, and

TABLE 4.

Comparison of Operative Results in Renal Artery Occlusion
(RA-OCC) and Renal Artery Stenosis *(RAS)* Groups

	RA-OCC (n = 95)	RAS (n = 302)	*P*-value
Perioperative mortality (%)	5.3	4.0	0.59
Hypertension response (%)			0.52
Cured	11	13	
Improved	80	74	
No change	9	13	
Renal function response (%)*			0.20
Improved	49	41	
No change/worsened	51	59	

*Preoperative serum creatinine ≥ 1.3 mg/dL.

TABLE 5.

Results of Proportional Hazards Regression Model of
Follow-up Survival for Patients With Renal Artery
Occlusion (n = 90)

Variable	Beta	Standard Error	Hazard Ratio	*P*-value
Increase in EGFR	−0.980	0.288	0.38	<0.01
Age	1.329	0.385	3.78	<0.01
Preoperative SCr	0.567	0.174	1.76	<0.01
History of CHF	1.296	0.530	3.66	0.01
Preoperative SBP	−0.159	0.091	0.85	0.08

Abbreviations: EGFR, estimated glomerular filtration rate; *SCr,* serum
creatinine; *CHF,* congestive heart failure; *SBP,* systolic blood pressure.

history of transient ischemic attack or stroke demonstrated significant and independent association with decreased survival (Table 6). The product-limit estimate of time to death in the RA-OCC group is depicted by a *solid line* in Figure 2.

On the basis of criteria previously described, the blood pressure response in the 90 patients surviving surgical repair for RA-OCC was considered cured in 10 (11%), improved in 72 (80%), and 8 (9%) were considered failed (Table 4). Beneficial blood pressure re-

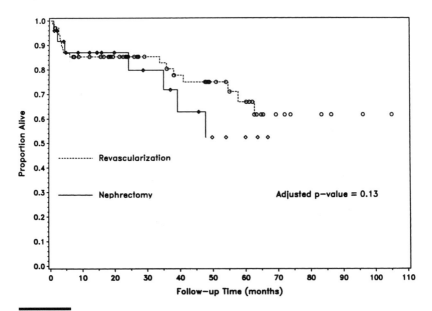

FIGURE 1.
Product-limit estimate of survival among patients with renal artery occlusion, by surgery type.

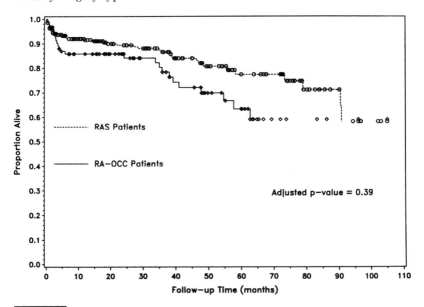

FIGURE 2.
Product-limit estimate of survival among renal artery occlusion *(RA-OCC)* and renal artery stenosis *(RAS)* patients.

TABLE 6.
Results of Proportional Hazards Regression Model of
Follow-up Survival for Patients With Atherosclerotic
Renovascular Disease (n = 380)

Variable	Beta	Standard Error	Hazard Ratio	P-value
RA-OCC	0.248	0.269	1.28	0.36
Age	0.921	0.185	2.51	<0.01
CHF	0.576	0.289	1.78	0.05
TIA/CVA	0.784	0.277	2.19	<0.01
Dialysis	−2.022	0.725	0.13	<0.01
Preoperative SCr	0.957	0.208	2.60	<0.01

Abbreviations: RA-OCC, renal artery occlusion; *CHF,* congestive heart failure; *TIA/CVA,* transient ischemic attack/cerebrovascular accident; *SCr,* serum creatinine.

sponse (cured or improved) was equivalent after nephrectomy and revascularization (87% and 92%, respectively; *P* = 0.54; Table 3).

Forty-nine percent of 79 patients had improved renal function, with a 20% or more increase in serum creatinine level, including 9 patients removed from dialysis dependence. Those patients who had improved renal function demonstrated a significant and independent increase in estimated survival (Fig 3) and dialysis-free survival (Fig 4). A significant increase in renal function was observed after revascularization and after nephrectomy for RA-OCC if contralateral revascularization was performed (Table VII). A significant increase in renal function was not observed after nephrectomy alone.

Preoperative renal length was 7.3 ± 1.4 cm (range, 4–10.4 cm) in the nephrectomy group and 8.2 ± 1.5cm (range, 5–12.2 cm) in the revascularized group (*P* = 0.01). Of 9 revascularized kidneys less than 7 cm in length, all had a beneficial blood pressure response and 4 (44%) had improved renal function. In comparison, 8 nephrectomies were performed on kidneys less than 7 cm in length. Beneficial blood pressure response was observed in 6 (75%), whereas 3 (38%) had improvement in excretory renal function. Renal length (9.0 ± 0.3 cm) after revascularization of RA-OCC in 31 kidneys was significantly increased (*P* = 0.04) compared with preoperative renal length (8.6 ± 0.3 cm).

Within the nephrectomy group, preoperative studies demonstrated a nephrogram in 5 of 22 kidneys (23%) compared with 49

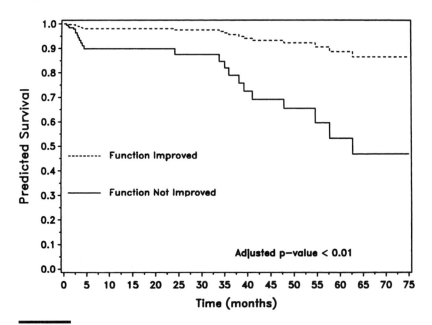

FIGURE 3.
Predicted survival for renal artery occlusion patients with improved or un-improved renal function after revascularization.

of 65 kidneys (75%) in the revascularized group ($P < 0.01$). Reconstitution of the distal renal artery was present in 8 of 21 kidneys (38%) in the nephrectomy group and 48 of 60 kidneys (80%) in the revascularized group ($P < 0.01$). While the absence of a nephrogram or distal reconstitution of the renal artery was significantly associated with nephrectomy in both cases, absence did not preclude revascularization in 48% of kidneys without nephrogram or distal renal artery reconstitution. In fact, 8 of 21 patients (38%) with neither preoperative nephrogram nor distal renal artery reconstitution underwent operative renal artery revascularization. Six of these eight patients (75%) had a beneficial blood pressure response, whereas six patients (75%) had improved renal function.

Comparisons were made between the 95 patients with RA-OCC and the 302 patients with RAS (Table 1). Patients with RA-OCC tended toward severe hypertension (mean systolic blood pressure, 204 ± 31 mm Hg vs. 197 ± 38 mm Hg; $P = 0.08$) requiring more antihypertensive medications (3.0 ± 1.1 drugs vs. 2.5 ± 1.1 drugs; $P < 0.01$), had more severe renal dysfunction (60% vs. 35%; $P < 0.01$), and more prevalent end-organ failure (congestive heart failure [34% vs. 16%; $P < 0.01$] and dialysis dependence [12% vs. 5%; $P =$

0.03]). During postoperative evaluation, 87% of patients in the RAS group had a beneficial blood pressure response compared with 91% of patients in the RA-OCC group ($P = 0.52$; Table 4). In the RAS group, 41% of patients had improved renal function compared with 49% of patients in the RA-OCC group ($P = 0.20$).

As a group, hypertensive patients with RA-OCC have a high rate of renal insufficiency (88%) and a high incidence of site-specific end-organ atherosclerotic disease (95%). Despite the presence of end-organ failure and extrarenal atherosclerosis, the perioperative mortality was equivalent for renal revascularization and nephrectomy. An equivalent beneficial blood pressure response was observed after both revascularization and nephrectomy (92% and 87%, respectively); however, only revascularization or revascularization with nephrectomy demonstrated a significant increase in estimated glomerular filtration rate. In comparison with the RAS patients, patients with RA-OCC had more severe hypertension, an increased prevalence of congestive heart failure, decreased renal excretory function, increased prevalence of preoperative dialysis dependence, and required bilateral revascularization more frequently. Despite these differences, perioperative mortality and the

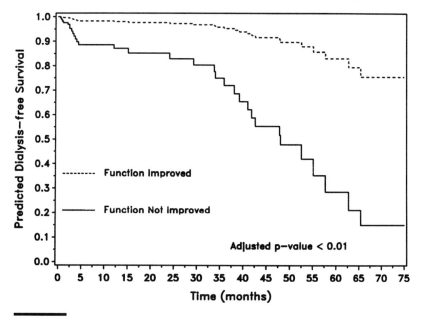

FIGURE 4.
Predicted dialysis-free survival for renal artery occlusion patients with improved or unimproved renal function after revascularization.

TABLE 7.

Change in Estimated Glomerular Filtration Rate (EGFR) of Renal Artery Occlusion Patients, by Site of Disease and Extent of Repair

	No. of Patients	Preoperative EGFR (Mean ± SE)		Postoperative EGFR (Mean ± SE)	Adjusted Postoperative EGFR (Mean ± SE)
Unilateral					
Nephrectomy	4	47.3 ± 9.1	←$P = 0.08$→	50.4 ± 8.4	36.3 ± 5.0
		↑ $P = 0.04$ ↓			↑ $P = 0.57$ ↓
Revascularization	21	29.6 ± 3.1	←$P < 0.01$→	36.8 ± 3.7	39.5 ± 2.1
Bilateral					
Nephrectomy	14	31.5 ± 3.2	←$P = 0.02$→	38.7 ± 4.6	34.8 ± 3.6
		↑ $P = 0.12$ ↓			↑ $P = 0.99$ ↓
Revascularization	40	25.6 ± 1.9	←$P < 0.01$→	33.5 ± 3.1	35.1 ± 2.1

follow-up survival were similar for patients treated for RA-OCC and RAS.

Because blood pressure response is equivalent after nephrectomy or revascularization, and improved renal function after renal artery repair appears to confer improved follow-up survival, our results support renal artery revascularization for RA-OCC. The practical value of this premise is obvious when one considers that as many as 35% of patients with mild contralateral occlusive lesions will progress to hemodynamically severe occlusive lesions within 5 years.[5] Once nephrectomy has been performed for renovascular hypertension and contralateral renal artery disease progresses, global renal function is threatened and operative intervention may be performed for severe renal insufficiency in the presence of a lesion that is no longer amenable to reconstruction. Conversely, overzealous revascularization of a poorly functioning or nonfunctioning kidney will sometimes lead to revascularization of a kidney in which no functional response can be achieved.

In an attempt to predict functional response to operation, the absence of distal renal artery reconstitution has been considered an indication for nephrectomy. Although absence of reconstitution does make revascularization less likely, 48% of such patients in our experience proved to have a patent distal renal artery on exploration. Subsequent revascularization in this setting was associated with beneficial blood pressure (85%) and renal function response (62%). The presence of a nephrogram has also been proposed as an indicator of operative outcome, but 48% of the patients without a nephrogram demonstrated by preoperative angiography were successfully revascularized in our experience. Renal length of less than 8–9 cm has been suggested as a predictor of poor postoperative renal functional response, but recent success has been found in revascularization of small kidneys.[8] Although our nephrectomy group did have a smaller renal size on average, we found that absolute renal length did not preclude revascularization, beneficial blood pressure response, or improved renal function after repair. Successful outcome was seen in patients with kidneys that could be deemed unsuitable for reconstruction based upon kidney length alone. Distal renal artery reconstitution, presence of a nephrogram, and renal length were associated with nephrectomy but did not preclude beneficial blood pressure or renal function response or patency of repair.

Although the kidney with RA-OCC may receive sufficient collateral flow to prevent infarction, RA-OCC is frequently associated with a decrease in size and changes in histology. Often there is tubular atrophy and hyalinization of glomeruli with a concomitant decrease in cortical thickness. Zinman and Libertino[9] found preoperative renal biopsy to be an indicator of functional response. While normal glomerular architecture supports retrieval of glomerular function, hyalinization does not preclude functional benefit because these histologic changes may be focal, and biopsy material may not be representative of the entire kidney.

SUMMARY

Patients with RA-OCC demonstrate equivalent blood pressure response after either revascularization or nephrectomy; however, only revascularization significantly improves excretory renal function. Because improved renal function is associated with improved estimated survival and the lower limits of renal function retrieval are not well defined, these results support renal revascularization in preference to nephrectomy for RA-OCC. We believe nephrectomy should be limited to patients with renovascular hypertension with an unreconstructable renal artery to a kidney with negligible excretory renal function. In this case, nephrectomy can provide benefit in control of hypertension without decreasing overall excretory renal function.

REFERENCES

1. Dean RH, Tribble RW, Hansen KJ, et al: Evolution of renal insufficiency in ischemic nephropathy. *Ann Surg* 213:446–455, 1991.
2. Hansen KJ, Thomason B, Craven TE, et al: Surgical management of dialysis-dependent ischemic nephropathy. *J Vasc Surg* 21:197–211, 1995.
3. Appel RG, Bleyer AJ, Reavis S, et al: Renovascular disease in older patients beginning renal replacement therapy. *Kidney Int* 48:171–176, 1995.
4. Dean RH, Kieffer RW, Smith BM, et al: Renovascular hypertension: Anatomic and renal function changes during drug therapy. *Arch Surg* 116:1408–1415, 1981.
5. Dean RH, Wilson JP, Burko H, et al: Saphenous vein aortorenal bypass grafts: Serial arteriographic study. *Ann Surg* 180:469–478, 1974.
6. Hansen KJ, Tribble RW, Reavis SW, et al: Renal duplex sonography: Evaluation of clinical utility. *J Vasc Surg* 12:227–236, 1990.
7. Oskin TC, Hansen KJ, Dietch JC, et al: Chronic renal artery occlusion: Nephrectomy vs. revascularization, submitted for publication.
8. Dean RH, Englund R, DuPont WD, et al: Retrieval of renal function by revascularization. *Ann Surg* 202:367–375, 1985.
9. Zinman LN, Libertino JA: Revascularization of the chronically occluded renal artery with restoration of renal function. *J Urol* 118:517–521, 1977.

PART IV

Upper Extremity Ischemia

CHAPTER 9

Current Management of the Ischemic Hand

Christian E. Sampson, M.D.
Instructor in Surgery, Harvard Medical School, Brigham and Women's Hospital, Boston, Massachusetts

Julian J. Pribaz, M.D.
Associate Professor of Surgery, Harvard Medical School, Brigham and Women's Hospital, Boston, Massachusetts

H and ischemia occurs infrequently and is present in only 5% of patients who have symptomatic extremity ischemia.[1] Despite its many causes, patients with hand ischemia have similar signs and symptoms. Cold intolerance—that is, pain or paresthesias in some or all the digits, or in the entire hand with exposure to cold—is very common. Ischemic rest pain does occur but is less prevalent in the hand or upper extremity than in the foot or lower extremity. Careful questioning may reveal a history of ischemic rest pain. Symptoms can often be elicited by simple provocative tests, such as repetitive clenching of the fist or raising the patients' arm over their head. Rest pain typically indicates occlusive disease in the subclavian or axillary arteries.

Patients may also have noticed color changes in their digits with exposure to cold or some other type of stress. Raynaud's phenomenon is characterized by sequential color changes of the digits starting with blanching, followed by cyanosis, and finally hyperemia, which can be associated with a painful burning type of dysesthesia. Raynaud's phenomenon is usually bilateral and is a manifestation of the final common vasospastic pathway seen in many connective tissue disorders. Unilateral Raynaud's phenomenon may be a vasospastic response to proximal, large-vessel occlusive disease or disease of the distal radial and/or ulnar arteries at the wrist.[2]

The specific cause of the vascular occlusion will, in general, correlate with the level of involvement. It may be caused by small or large vessel pathology, and lead to acute or chronic ischemia of the hand or digits. The most common cause is embolization from a cardiac source, but emboli may also originate from ulcerated atheromatous plaques in proximal large vessels caused by organic arterial stenoses and occlusions.[3] The clinical manifestations of distal embolization depend upon the size of the emboli. Microemboli may cause splinter hemorrhages of the nail beds. Larger emboli will be associated with a spectrum of ischemic manifestations, from small digital tip ulcerations caused by occlusion of the distal segment of a digital artery, to ischemia of the entire hand and distal forearm seen with brachial artery occlusion at the bifurcation of the radial and ulnar arteries.

The management of patients with an ischemic hand as the result of trauma or iatrogenic injury is generally straightforward. This chapter will concentrate on the diagnosis and management of patients with ischemia as a manifestation of systemic disease.

ETIOLOGY

Table 1 lists some of the conditions that can cause acute or chronic ischemia of the digits or hand. Jones[4] has outlined four pathophysiologic mechanisms intrinsic to the arterial system itself that can produce ischemia: embolization, thrombosis, arteriosclerosis, and vasospasm. Any one of these will lead to a reduction of arterial flow below that needed to meet the basal metabolic demands of the upper extremity. In comparison, extrinsic causes are rare and occur when ischemia is produced by direct arterial compression or interruption as occurs in thoracic outlet syndrome, supracondylar fracture of the humerus, shoulder dislocation, posterior elbow dislocation, blunt trauma producing a compartment syndrome, or iatrogenic, accidental, or deliberate penetrating trauma. These problems are, in most cases, easily recognizable and treatment is clear-cut. They will therefore not be discussed further.

EMBOLI

Embolization to the upper extremity is the most common cause of hand ischemia. The condition is easily recognized by the classic signs and symptoms known as the "five P's": pain, pallor, pulselessness, paresthesias, and paralysis.[5] The heart is the most common source of emboli, which are typically seen after myocardial infarction or associated with atrial fibrillation. Such emboli often lodge at the bifurcation of the brachial artery, producing acute ischemia of the forearm and hand. Anyone with upper extremity embolization will often have a history of significant cardiac disease and/or other

TABLE 1.
Etiology of Acute and Chronic Ischemia of the Hand and Digits

Emboli
    Atrial fibrillation
    Myocardial infarction
    Poststenotic dilatation of proximal vessels
    Atherosclerotic ulcerated plaque of proximal vessels
Atherosclerosis of subclavian and axillary arteries
Trauma
    Shoulder dislocation
    Supracondylar fracture of the humerus
    Posterior dislocation of the elbow
    Ulnar artery thrombosis (hypothenar hammer syndrome)
    Blunt or penetrating trauma to digits, hand, forearm, or upper arm
Thoracic outlet syndrome
    Scalene muscle compression
    Cervical or first rib compression
Iatrogenic
    Brachial artery catheterization
    Radial artery—arterial pressure cannulation
Arteriovenous fistulas
    Dialysis access
    Posttraumatic
Intra-arterial drug injections
Connective tissue disorders
    Scleroderma
    Systemic lupus erythematosus
    Rheumatoid arthritis
    Mixed connective tissue disease
    Wegener's granulomatosis
Renal vascular disease
Fibromuscular dysplasia
Buerger's disease
Hematologic disorders
    Polycythemia vera
    Leukemia
    Myeloma
    Cryoglobulinemia
Vibratory tool disease
Postirradiation
Septicemia
Malignancy

medical conditions. Thus, it is important to remember that embolism or thrombosis of the upper extremity caused by associated underlying disease has a poor prognosis, with significant morbidity in the first 2 years after therapy.[6] One study showed a 1-year patient survival rate of 29% and 50% for medical and surgical therapy, respectively, after embolization to the upper extremity.[7]

As mentioned earlier, the level of ischemia caused by embolization depends upon the size of the emboli. More distal ischemia can result from a shower of microemboli emanating from a number of potential sources including proximal atherosclerotic plaques, aneurysms, mural thrombi resulting from thoracic outlet syndrome, or from the heart. These are seen as splinter hemorrhages in the nail beds or as digital tip ulcerations. However, the condition can be more severe, with ischemia involving entire digits or the entire hand and forearm depending upon the level of arterial occlusion.

THROMBOSIS

Arterial thrombosis can be either local or diffuse. The classic case of localized thrombosis producing hand ischemia, albeit rare, is the "hypothenar hammer syndrome."[8] This syndrome is characterized by thrombosis of the ulnar artery and superficial palmar arch caused by repetitive trauma of the vessel against the hook of the hamate bone. It is typically seen in individuals whose occupation promotes the use of the ulnar border of their hand as a hammer. Von Rosen,[9] in discussing this type of problem involving the ulnar artery, postulated that intimal damage would lead to thrombosis, whereas damage of the media would lead to true aneurysm formation. Thrombosis can also occasionally occur after brachial artery catheterization or radial artery cannulation. The rate of complications causing hand ischemia after cardiac catheterization via the brachial artery has been reported to be as low as 0.57%.[10] Radial artery cannulation causes problems more frequently as shown by Crossland and Neviaser who reported a 10% incidence of hand or digital ischemia which, in some cases, led to loss of digits.[11]

More devastating is diffuse thrombosis of hand and digital arteries. This is most often seen after localized intra-arterial drug injections, or secondary to the disseminated intravascular coagulation associated with infections, particularly meningococcemia (purpura fulminans), and malignancies.

ARTERIAL DISEASE

Intimal thickening with accumulation of cellular and noncellular elements leading to progressive occlusion and calcification is seen in atherosclerosis, Buerger's disease (thrombangitis obliterans), and renal vascular disease. Thrombangitis obliterans commonly causes upper extremity ischemia, with one study reporting a 26% incidence of upper and lower extremity ischemia combined, and a 28% incidence of upper extremity ischemia alone.[12] The arterial calcification present in patients with advanced atherosclerotic disease may easily be visible on a plain radiograph. Some patients may have an accelerated atherosclerotic process resulting from the effects of long-standing subclinical microemboli. The vasculature of patients with collagen vascular disorders may show a variety of pathologic changes including intimal hyperplasia and fibrosis, which cause ischemic symptoms.[13] Patients with chronic renal failure are placed in double jeopardy because not only does their abnormal calcium metabolism, causing hypercalcemia and calciphylaxis, lead to accelerated arteriosclerosis, but creation of an arteriovenous fistula for hemodialysis can produce ischemia via a steal effect or embolization.[14, 15] Fibromuscular dysplasia with media hyperplasia, although not an arteriosclerotic process, is included here as an unusual cause of hand ischemia.[16]

VASOSPASM

Increased sympathetic activity or tone, causing a reduction of blood flow, is the presumed mechanism of ischemia in patients with Raynaud's disease or the Raynaud's phenomenon associated with connective tissue disorders, such as scleroderma or systemic lupus erythematosus. Specific criteria have been established to separate Raynaud's disease from Raynaud's phenomenon, which is characterized by intermittent signs and symptoms of ischemia caused by an underlying systemic condition. The following criteria are used for diagnosing primary Raynaud's disease: (1) characteristic color changes—white to blue to red—induced by exposure to cold or stress; (2) bilateral hand involvement; (3) no arterial occlusion proximal to the fingers; (4) absence of gangrene or trophic changes except at the very tips of the fingers; (5) absence of underlying disease that may cause vasomotor problems, especially connective tissue disorders; (6) symptoms present for greater than 2 years; and (7) occurrence predominantly in female patients.[17] Two years without signs and symptoms of a systemic disorder may not be long enough to rule out Raynaud's phenomenon. It is now known that many patients with Raynaud's disease, if followed long enough, will be diagnosed with a connective tissue disease with secondary Raynaud's phenomenon.

In one series, the interval between Raynaud's symptoms and the diagnosis of connective tissue disease averaged 11.5 years, ranging from 3 to 16 years.[18] In addition, as immunologic testing methods have become more sophisticated, patients with Raynaud's disease are having their diagnosis changed to Raynaud's phenomenon. To avoid confusion, there is now general acceptance of the term Raynaud's syndrome for all patients whether or not there is an underlying disease to explain the symptoms and that the terms "Raynaud's disease" and "Raynaud's phenomenon" should not be used. Therefore, "Raynaud's syndrome" will be used exclusively in the remainder of this chapter. It is clear that sympathetic overactivity and progressive occlusion of the digital arteries are responsible for the characteristic changes seen in Raynaud's patients, but the debate continues as to which occurs first. It has been suggested that increased sympathetic activity may be either the result of, or actually cause, local arterial disease or occlusion. That is, autonomically induced vasospasm can, over time, cause segmental occlusions of the digital arteries.[19–21]

DIAGNOSIS

As mentioned earlier, acute ischemia is easily recognized and diagnosed, and specific therapy is clear-cut. Chronic ischemic signs and symptoms are more challenging. It is important to obtain a careful history and perform a thorough physical examination. The interview and examination should take place in a well-lighted, warm room. A cold room—indeed, merely being in a doctor's office—can induce peripheral vasospasm, severely limiting a thorough examination. Wherever the examination is performed, the patient should be made to feel as relaxed and comfortable as possible. Medical risk factors should be noted, especially the presence of insulin-dependent diabetes and hypercholesterolemia, as well as a history of myocardial infarction or arrhythmia, renal disease, or peripheral vascular disease of the lower extremities. Current medications with any vasoactive potential are noted. Current and past tobacco use is of obvious importance. A systematic examination of the upper extremity is then performed. If there is evidence to support a diagnosis of proximal arterial pathology or a connective tissue disorder, then appropriate consultations are made to a vascular surgeon or rheumatologist, respectively. Particular attention should be paid to the frequency, duration, and time of symptoms noticed by the patient. In cases of Raynaud's syndrome, there is often seasonal variation, with symptoms worse in the fall and winter. Patients must be asked about previous trauma or surgery, with particular attention paid to the location of scars.

A sensory and motor examination of each hand must be performed, including digital two-point and light touch discrimination, intrinsic muscle strength, and overall grip strength. The temperature and color of the hand and the digits should be noted, as well as whether the palms are moist or dry. The hands and fingers are examined for trophic changes, ulcerations, blisters, and periungual changes. Patients with chronic ischemia may have a peculiar subungual thickening, and many of these patients will have an underlying connective tissue disorder such as scleroderma or lupus erythematosus.

DOPPLER EXAMINATION AND ALLEN'S TEST

The modified Allen's test is the quickest way to determine the contribution of the radial and ulnar arteries to digital and hand blood flow via an intact superficial palmar arch. The radial and ulnar arteries are occluded at the wrist after the patient makes a clenched fist. The examiner then notes the time required for capillary refill in the hand after releasing each artery. The test is considered positive—that is, presence of an incomplete superficial arch—if capillary refill takes longer than 3 seconds. A pulse oximeter applied to the fingers can be used in lieu of visually assessing capillary refill. Finally, a "digital artery" Allen's test may provide useful information about adequacy of blood flow in the digital arteries. It is performed by exsanguinating the digit by asking the patient to actively flex the finger. The examiner then compresses both digital arteries, and the patient then gently extends the finger. The radial digital artery is then released, maintaining pressure on the ulnar digital artery, and capillary refill time noted. The procedure is then repeated with release of the ulnar digital artery while maintaining pressure on the radial digital artery.

Palpation of pulses is performed in each extremity beginning with the subclavian artery and proceeding to the brachial, radial (including the dorsal branch in the anatomical snuff box), and ulnar arteries. The clavicular area should be auscultated for the presence of a bruit. Segmental blood pressures should be obtained in each arm. A difference of 20 mm Hg between the brachial artery and the distal radial and ulnar arteries in the same extremity or either arm at the same level is significant.

Continuous wave (CW) Doppler examination of the radial and ulnar arteries is performed, and the "signal" traced as far distal as possible, including the anatomical snuff box, the hypothenar region, and superficial palmar arch. It is important to realize that CW Doppler cannot differentiate the superficial and deep palmar arches. It is therefore impossible to distinguish a thrombosed (or absent) superficial arch from a patent deep arch with CW Doppler. It may also be difficult to isolate the common digital arteries, but an attempt at mapping these should be made. The proper digital arteries are easily and accurately assessed with the CW Doppler ultrasound, and should be followed out the length of each digit for both the radial and ulnar vessels. If the signal is lost, the level at which it is lost should be noted. Duplex ultrasound machines are available in most non-invasive vascular laboratories and can provide more information about the arterial anatomy, including sites of narrowing or occlusion, anatomical variations in particular patients, and flow rates. Use and interpretation of duplex ultrasound requires expertise, but if available it is the noninvasive procedure of choice. Because CW Doppler is generally more readily available and easier to use, it remains a valuable adjunct in the initial patient assessment.

PLETHYSMOGRAPHY
Digital plethysmography with digital pressure cuffs can be used to obtain objective data (blood pressure) and a qualitative assessment (waveform analysis) of the blood flow in each finger. A difference in pressure of 15 mm Hg between fingers or 30 mm Hg between a finger and the pressure at the level of the radial and ulnar arteries in the wrist is indicative of occlusion or stenosis at or distal to the palmar arches. The normal waveform of blood flow in the digital arteries, as elsewhere, shows a sharp upstroke with a dicrotic notch on the downslope. Reduced flow will be seen as a flattened and broadened curve without a dicrotic notch. In patients who require surgery, digital plethysmography is useful to compare postoperative results with the preoperative state.

COLD STRESS TESTING
Cold stress testing as described by Koman et al.,[22] is a more involved procedure used to study those patients whose symptoms were presumed to be caused by vasospastic disease in the hand and determining the effect of surgical sympathectomy.

The patients studied had painful ulcerated digits unresponsive to medical therapy, Raynaud's syndrome secondary to a connective tissue disorder, or nonreconstructible lesions based on arteriography. Patients with occlusive or embolic lesions above the proximal forearm were excluded. With digital temperature and laser Doppler flow monitoring, the hand is cooled to 10°C for 20 minutes and then rewarmed. Symptomatic vascular insufficiency is re-

Subscribe to the related journal in your field!

Yes! Begin my one-year subscription to
Journal of Vascular Surgery (12 issues).

Name _____

Institution _____

Address _____

City _____ State _____

ZIP/PC _____ Country _____

Specialty _____
(Students/residents, please list Institution)

Subscription prices (through 9/30/98)

		USA	Canada*	Int'l
Individuals	❑	$148.00	$196.88	$184.00
Institutions	❑	279.00	337.05	315.00
Students, residents	❑	74.00	117.70	110.00

Method of payment

Enclose payment (check or credit card number)
and we'll send an extra issue FREE!

❑ **Check** (in U.S. dollars, drawn on a U.S. bank, and
payable to *Journal of Vascular Surgery*)

❑ VISA ❑ MasterCard ❑ Discover

❑ AmEx ❑ Bill me Exp. date_____

Card #_____

Signature _____

*Includes Canadian GST

Individual/student subscriptions must be in the name of,
billed to, and paid for by the individual.

Airmail rates available upon request.
Prices subject to change without notice.

J024983YC

Reservation Card for Advances

Yes! I would like my own copy of *Advances in Vascular Surgery*® at the price of **$81.00** plus sales
tax, postage, and handling. Please begin my subscription with the current edition according to the
terms described below.* I understand that I will have 30 days to examine each annual edition.

Name _____

Address _____

City _____ State _____ ZIP_____

Method of Payment

Check (in U.S. dollars, drawn on a U.S. bank, payable to *Advances in Vascular Surgery*®)

❑ VISA ❑ MasterCard ❑ Discover ❑ AmEx ❑ Bill me

Card number _____ Exp. date: _____

Signature _____

Prices are subject to change without notice. PMC-043

---

*Your Advances service guarantee:

When you subscribe to *Advances*, you will receive advance notice of future annual volumes about
two months before publication. To receive the new edition, you need do nothing—we'll send you
the new volume as soon as it is available. If you want to discontinue, the advance notice allows you
time to notify us of your decision. If you are not completely satisfied, you have 30 days to return
any *Advances*.

BUSINESS REPLY MAIL
FIRST-CLASS MAIL   PERMIT NO 135   ST LOUIS MO

POSTAGE WILL BE PAID BY ADDRESSEE

SUBSCRIPTION SERVICES
MOSBY–YEAR BOOK, INC.
11830 WESTLINE INDUSTRIAL DRIVE
ST. LOUIS   MO 63146-9988

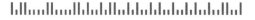

BUSINESS REPLY MAIL
FIRST-CLASS MAIL   PERMIT NO 135   ST LOUIS MO

POSTAGE WILL BE PAID BY ADDRESSEE

M Mosby

PAT NEWMAN
11830 WESTLINE INDUSTRIAL DRIVE
PO BOX 46908
ST. LOUIS   MO 63146-9934

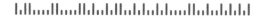

Want to speed up the process?

To order the *Advances*, you also
may call 1-800-426-4545

To subscribe to the journal today,
call toll-free in the U.S.:
1-800-453-4351
or fax 314-432-1158
Outside the U.S., call: 314-453-4351

Visit us at:
www.mosby.com/Mosby/Periodicals

Mosby–Year Book, Inc.
Subscription Services
11830 Westline Industrial Drive
St. Louis, MO 63146 U.S.A.

M Mosby

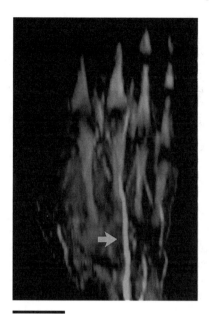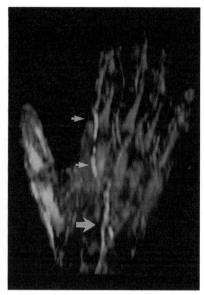

FIGURE 1.
Left: preop MRA. Right: postop MRA. Large arrows: ulnar artery. Small arrows: vein graft.

vealed by abnormal baseline, cooling, and rewarming temperature and arterial flow vs. time curves compared to normal controls. Arterial flow was measured by laser Doppler.

A modification of this is to monitor cold recovery time from immersion of the hand in a 60°F water bath.[23] Wilgis[24] has used cold stress testing with and without local sympathetic blockade, by performing a digital block with lidocaine, to identify those patients whose symptoms are caused by reversible vasospasm. Digital sympathectomy would be offered to those patients whose abnormal cold stress test results were normalized by the digital block. However, our experience, and results shown by others,[25] is that even nonresponders may benefit from surgical sympathectomy.

ARTERIOGRAPHY
Magnetic resonance angiography (MRA) is a noninvasive technique that offers acceptable resolution and has the advantage of providing oblique, cross-sectional, and longitudinal views of the fingers and hand. It has a lower morbidity and lower cost than conventional angiography. Figure 1 shows a preoperative and postoperative MRA in a patient with an allergy to IV contrast who had a pain-

ful, ischemic index finger. The preoperative MRA was able to demonstrate a lesion at the level of the common digital artery amenable to bypass. The patient underwent a reversed vein bypass procedure from the ulnar artery to the radial proper digital artery with complete resolution of her ischemia. The postoperative MRA shows the vein graft to be open with improved distal flow. As more centers gain experience and refine this technique, it may replace routine angiography and become the anatomical study of choice. Some are using this as a first-line tool when investigating purely vasospastic disorders because there is no induced vasospasm and excellent resolution.[23]

However, for the present, conventional angiography or digital subtraction angiography remains the gold standard for evaluating arterial pathology despite several drawbacks. They are more costly and invasive, have a higher incidence of complications, and on rare occasions will lead the clinician to a false conclusion because of contrast-induced arterial spasm. Contrast agent–induced spasm can be eliminated or mitigated by concurrent administration of vasodilating agents such as nitroglycerin, nifedipine, or tolazoline. Some centers recommend performing an axillary block for sympathetic blockade before angiography when a vasospastic disorder is suspected as the underlying pathology. Conventional angiography should be performed via the femoral artery, not the brachial artery, and the entire upper extremity evaluated including the aortic arch. Intraluminal filling defects as opposed to fixed areas of stenosis suggest the possibility of microembolization from a proximal source. In the hand, the physician should look for the presence of complete superficial and deep arches, three common digital arteries to the second, third and fourth web spaces, and radial and ulnar proper digital arteries to each finger. Absence of one or more common digital artery implies a problem at the level of the superficial arch. If there is no evidence of arterial obstruction either before or after administration of a vasodilating agent such as tolazoline, it can safely be assumed that vasospasm is the predominant mechanism responsible for the patient's ischemic symptoms.

Clearly not every patient with hand ischemia requires an angiogram, but one should be obtained when the following conditions are present: (1) unilateral Raynaud's syndrome, (2) progressive or recurrent digital gangrene despite maximal medical management, and (3) Doppler evidence of occlusion of a major artery. Whether performing MRA or conventional angiography, the study should include magnification views for improved detail of the common and proper digital arteries. In interpreting the study, the dynamic filling phase of the study must be reviewed, in addition to the static images. This will provide valuable information regarding sites causing a significant reduction in flow not readily apparent on the static images. Areas suggestive of reversible spasm may be identified by the intra-arterial administration of one of the vasodilating agents mentioned above.

OTHER METHODS

Other methods available to evaluate arterial flow include laser Doppler, thermography, and nuclear scans. Thermography and nuclear scans do not offer a significant advantage over CW or duplex Doppler ultrasound examination, and most likely they will soon be of historic interest only. The laser Doppler is a very sensitive device but because of its high cost, it has not gained a foothold in clinical practice and remains useful primarily as a laboratory tool. The latest generation duplex Doppler ultrasound machines offer high-resolution intraoperative use. They clearly offer the surgeon the ability to identify potential problems with direct revascularization procedures before closure, and may be of use in assessing the immediate effects of sympathectomy on digital blood flow.

At our institution, CW and duplex Doppler ultrasound examination, arteriography, and digital plethysmography with or without cold stress testing are the predominant methods of preoperative and postoperative assessment. Currently, MRA is used if there is a specific contraindication to conventional angiography.

MANAGEMENT

EMBOLECTOMY

In the absence of trauma, an acute episode of hand or digital ischemia is most often caused by arterial embolization. The diagnosis is easily confirmed by arteriography. Embolectomy is best used for localized lesions without evidence of diffuse distal thrombosis, and in conditions of severe limb-threatening ischemia with motor-sensory loss. Having said this, the procedure should only be considered if the patient's overall medical condition will permit a surgical procedure. Systemic heparinization is usually indicated, either before or after the arteriography. Occasionally the arteriogram will demonstrate a proximal arterial source of the emboli. In these cases a vascular surgeon will address both the emboli and the source at the same time. If no proximal arterial pathology is identified, and the embolus appears to be in one of the forearm vessels, then a standard embolectomy procedure via the brachial artery at the bifurcation is planned. Surgical embolectomy may be combined with intra-arterial thrombolytic therapy.

Occasionally, when embolization of the superficial palmar arch has occurred, embolectomy can be performed via the radial and/or ulnar arteries at the wrist level with a 1- or 2-mm catheter. This requires a very precise arteriotomy and subsequent repair to minimize arterial damage and stenosis at this level. Thrombolytic therapy may be used for incomplete or unsuccessful embolectomy. Streptokinase, or most commonly, urokinase may be used. In cases of persistent total occlusion, proximal inflow is occluded and 35,000–100,00 units of urokinase are infused and left for 20–30 minutes. Some cases warrant leaving the catheter in place for constant infusion of the thrombolytic agent for 1–3 days, with angiographic assessment every 24 hours. These patients require systemic heparinization to prevent thrombus formation around the indwelling catheter. Finally, there are new suction embolectomy devices available for the small vessels of the upper extremity which may gain in popularity. After embolectomy it is important to obtain an angiogram to document restoration of distal flow.

After successful embolectomy it is reasonable to keep the patient systemically heparinized for 5–7 days, followed by coumadin therapy for 3–6 months. After restitution of inflow, the patient should be monitored for the development of a compartment syndrome in the hand and/or forearm.

THROMBOLYTIC THERAPY

Indications for thrombolytic therapy are (1) delayed presentation after embolization where surgical embolectomy is unlikely to be unsuccessful because of intimal adherence of the embolus; (2) thrombosis caused by low flow from atherosclerotic disease[6] or intra-arterial injection[26]; and (3) cases where surgical embolectomy cannot be safely performed because of a patient's poor medical condition.

Thrombolytic agents available include streptokinase or urokinase (plasminogen activators) and recombinant tissue plasminogen activator (rt-PA).[6] Urokinase is the most commonly used thrombolytic agent.

Administration of the agent is via an arterial catheter maneuvered into position just proximal to the thrombus. The dosage of urokinase administered is 75,000–100,000 units/hr. Patients are given heparin intravenously to prevent pericatheter thrombosis. Duration of thrombolytic therapy may be from 10 to 93 hours.[6] Patients generally require monitoring in an ICU, with one or more returns to the angiography suite each day to assess progress. With complete lysis of a thrombus, a contrast study will delineate the arterial anatomy distal to the thrombus and may reveal the presence of a lesion responsible for the thrombosis. Such lesions are occasionally amenable to intervention in the angiography suite via balloon dilatation or possibly placement of an expandable stent. Surgery may be indicated if such intervention is not possible.

Results of upper extremity thrombolytic therapy are good, with limb salvage in all patients.[6, 27] Bleeding complications are the major concern with this type of therapy. Patients must be closely monitored for development of a groin or arm hematoma, or a cerebrovascular accident. One study of patients who underwent either upper or lower extremity intra-arterial thrombolytic therapy reported a 43.5% complication rate and a 5% mortality rate.[28] The majority of the deaths resulted from bleeding. Only one death was caused by myocardial infarction, but the fact remains that many of these patients have significant cardiovascular disease and mortality after thrombosis or embolism of the upper extremity.

Thrombolytic therapy has been used to treat subclavian artery thrombosis resulting from thoracic outlet syndrome,[29] and distal ulnar artery/proximal superficial palmar occlusion resulting from aneurysm formation with subsequent thrombosis (hypothenar hammer syndrome).[30] Although flow may be restored, the surgeon must be prepared to treat any underlying arterial pathology revealed, including the use of bypass grafts as there otherwise would be a high incidence of recurrent thrombosis. In the specific case of hypothenar hammer syndrome, our preference is to perform resection of the aneurysmal portions of the ulnar artery and arch, and reconstruction with a reversed forearm vein graft.

SYMPATHECTOMY

Sympathectomy may be either medical or surgical and, in general, is applied to two distinct patient populations. Surgical sympathectomy may be performed proximally or distally. One group of patients with hand or digital ischemia is found in the ICU; their ischemia is usually caused by the presence of a radial artery catheter for blood pressure monitoring. If these patients fail to improve with removal of the catheter, they may benefit from a medical sympathectomy by performing an axillary block with bupivicaine, the local anesthetic most often used.[31] The bupivicaine may be administered as a single bolus or as a continuous infusion via a catheter placed within the axillary sheath. The latter is preferable for the duration of therapy it offers, because clot dissolution or lysis may require several days to occur. Systemic anticoagulation is a contra-indication to performance of an axillary block because of the risk of hemorrhage into the axillary sheath, but once the catheter is in place anticoagulation is generally safe. If there is critical ischemia with loss of distal pulses and sensation, and no capillary refill, then an angiogram must be performed. Depending upon the findings, embolectomy, thrombolysis, or surgical intervention may be re-quired.

The other group of patients will have nonbypassable vascular disease, and many of these will have Raynaud's syndrome or hy-perhidrosis. These patients may be candidates for surgical sympa-thectomy. Hyperhidrosis has been treated with reasonable results via a thoracic (i.e., proximal) sympathectomy, now performed with minimally invasive endoscopic techniques.

The role of distal sympathectomy for the treatment of digital ischemia, with or without tip ulcerations, is more controversial. There are no long-term, prospective, blinded studies presenting ob-jective data to support its use. However, there is no doubt that prop-erly selected patients benefit from the procedure, with improved blood flow,[32] healing of ulcerations, and resolution of pain. Candi-dates for surgery are typically those who, despite maximal medi-cal therapy, have ongoing pain and ulcerations. The procedure in-cludes periadventital stripping, under high-power magnification, at several levels in the hand, including the distal radial and ulnar arteries, and the superficial arch, including the common digital ar-teries (Fig 2) and the proper digital arteries.[32] The procedure may be combined with a microsurgical revascularization procedure for even better results.[4, 33]

ARTERIAL BYPASS

Vascular bypass procedures in the upper extremity distal to the wrist are uncommon, and only recently have they been reported in the literature. There are two primary reasons such bypass pro-cedures are not as common as those performed in the lower ex-tremity: (1) the pattern of arteriosclerosis in the upper extremity does not lend itself to successful treatment with bypass procedures because of the distal extent of disease with poor runoff, and (2) there are technical difficulties in performing the bypass because of the small caliber of the vessels involved. Many patients will have calcified vessels and a paucity of suitable veins to select from for use as bypass conduits. Despite these inherent difficulties, a well-performed bypass procedure in the occasional patient with mid-

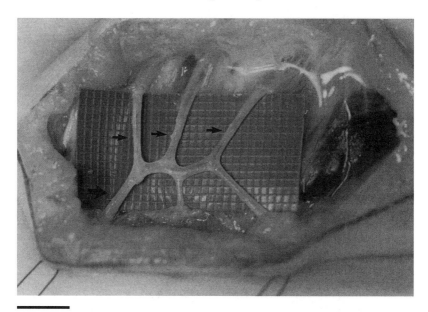

FIGURE 2.
Palmar sympathectomy. Large arrow: palmar arch. Small arrows: common digital arteries.

forearm to distal forearm occlusive disease can mean the difference between preserving a functional hand and amputation.

Two techniques using autogenous vein are available. A reversed segment of vein from the upper or lower extremity may be used as the conduit for the bypass procedure. Saphenous vein is better for bypassing lesions between the elbow and wrist, whereas an arm vein is a better size match for bypassing across or distal to the wrist. In some patients, especially in those with distal disease, the size mismatch between artery and reversed vein will make construction of an adequate anastomosis difficult. In these cases the surgeon should consider the other available technique, namely, in situ vein bypass. This perhaps should be considered the procedure of choice because it offers the best size match especially for bypass to the palmar arch or common digital vessels, minimizes endothelial trauma, and there is less likelihood of kinking with arm movement. The technique is technically more challenging, and sometimes a segment of vein must be procured from a distant site to obtain sufficient length. This is sometimes the case in patients with renal disease who have had prior dialysis access procedures, rendering unavailable the basilic and/or the cephalic veins. If additional vein is needed, it can be used in nonreversed fashion after ablating the valves.

In performing an in situ bypass, the vein must be completely exposed and all branches identified and ligated or clipped. The proximal anastomosis should be end-to-side to the distal brachial artery in the antecubital fossa. This is usually distal to the elbow flexion crease so that there will be no kinking of the graft with elbow flexion. The site for the distal anastomosis is planned using information from the preoperative angiogram to improve flow to the greatest amount of tissue possible. This will sometimes require performing more than one distal anastomosis by using a naturally occuring bifurcation of the vein, or constructing a "Y" with a small segment of vein anastomosed end-to-side to the main vein. This may be the case whether performing an in situ or reversed vein bypass. The distal anastomosis may be at the level of the common digital or even the proper digital arteries.

With in situ vein grafts, the objective is to ligate all branches while leaving the vein in its soft-tissue bed, because this offers the theoretical advantage of minimizing the potentially damaging effects of vein mobilization on the endothelial lining. A reverse-cutting valvulotome is passed from distal to proximal, and the valve leaflets of each valve are cut. The vein conduit is flushed with heparinized saline or lactated Ringer's solution, and checked for leaks or missed valves if the in situ technique is used. Repairs are made with 8-0 or 9-0 nylon. The proximal anastomosis is constructed first in standard end-to-side fashion. The patient should be systemically heparinized if an in situ vein is used, to prevent thrombosis at the sites of valve ablation. For reversed vein bypasses, intraoperative heparin should be used before arterial occlusion, but it does not need to be continued into the postoperative period. Once adequate flow in the graft is verified, distal anastomoses are performed. Here, the operating microscope offers the light and magnification necessary to perform anastomoses that may be as small as 1–2 mm. Occasionally, the arterial wall is too calcified to allow passage of the suture needle. In these cases a "sleeve" anastomosis technique can be helpful.[34] Using a double-armed 6-0 prolene stitch, two mattress stitches are placed 180 degrees apart, inside-out on both the vein and artery. The vein is then pulled, i.e., "sleeved," into the arterial lumen and the sutures tied.

Compared with lower extremity revascularization, there are few published reports on distal bypass procedures for upper extremity ischemia using reversed vein grafts. Those available, however, do support their use as an effective treatment modality.[35, 36] Nehler et al.[37] reported results of 17 distal bypass procedures in 15 patients, 5 with hand ischemia caused by arteriosclerotic complications from renal disease. Sixteen of 17 grafts, and all grafts performed for arteriosclerotic occlusive disease, remained patent at a mean follow-up of 14 months. However, two of the five patients with renal disease died of complications of their disease during the follow-up period. Clinical reports of in situ venous bypass procedures have also shown good results.[38] Ristow et al.[39] demonstrated excellent early and late results with in situ bypass for chronic severe ischemia in five patients; however, none of their patients had arteriosclerotic disease. Another earlier study of in situ bypass procedures included two patients with arteriosclerotic disease.[40] One in situ graft failed in one of the patients with arteriosclerotic disease because of poor runoff.

In treating chronic ischemia of the hand with revascularization procedures, the surgeon should consider performing a concomitant periadventitial sympathectomy.[39] As stated earlier, there are no long-term studies confirming the benefits of distal sympathectomy procedures, but there are data to support its use.[32] Therefore, concomitant distal sympathectomy should be considered because it adds little morbidity to direct revascularization procedures.

ARTERIOVENOUS REVERSAL

In patients with extensive distal disease and poor runoff, arterial reconstruction may not be possible. These patients may be candidates for arteriovenous reversal—that is, arterialization of the venous system with perfusion of the capillary beds by reversal of flow through the veins. A suitable in situ vein is selected and a valvulotomy performed, followed by proximal anastomosis to a major patent artery with no distal anastomoses performed. Studies in lower extremity animal models have shown that the procedure promotes neovascularization[41] and improved tissue perfusion.[42] A clinical study in six patients conducted by King et al.[47] showed limb salvage in all patients and symptomatic improvement in five. Two patients in this group had significant edema, and in one patient the arterialized vein thrombosed. This technique should be considered an investigational procedure and, until more study is done, should be used only in carefully selected patients by surgeons experienced with the technique.

OMENTAL TRANSFER

In patients who are not candidates for either revascularization or arteriovenous reversal, revascularization by free tissue transfer should be considered. The omentum has been used to revascularize the ischemic extremity both as a free and pedicled flap.[43, 44] A pedicled omental flap, with later division of the pedicle, has been used to revascularize an ischemic upper extremity.[45]

More recently, Pederson and Pribaz[46] have demonstrated the value of free omental transfer in the treatment of chronic upper extremity ischemia, and they make several points regarding successful use of this technique. Prerequisites for the procedure are suitable proximal vessels to provide inflow, and the patient must obviously have an adequate omentum. Patients with multiple abdominal procedures may not be good candidates because they may have dense adhesions present. The gastroepiploic vessels are generally of adequate quality for performing an anastomosis. Once the anastomoses have been performed, the omentum is either buried beneath skin flaps or covered by split-thickness skin grafts. Their results showed with rest pain subsides and ulcerations heal by 6 weeks after the procedure. Doppler signals over distal native vessels have returned in some patients. As is true for arteriovenous reversal, the procedure is relatively new and, although short-term results are promising, long-term benefit is not known. Therefore the procedure should only be offered to carefully selected patients.

AMPUTATION

Despite attempts to treat ischemia, irreversible tissue loss may occur. This often results in dry gangrene of variable length of a digit. In some cases it is reasonable to allow autoamputation to occur. This generally maximizes the final length of the digit. However, if the patient has significant pain or if there is concern an infection may develop, formal surgical amputation may be offered. At the level of the digits, this may be performed under local anesthesia. Equal-length palmar and dorsal flaps are planned, with the margins curved proximally to minimize "dog-ears." The neurovascular bundles must be identified to allow cauterization or ligation of the arteries. The nerves are cut sharply under tension to allow proximal retraction into the stump to prevent a painful neuroma from developing.

REFERENCES

1. McLafferty RB, Edwards JM, Taylor LM Jr, et al: Diagnosis and long-term clinical outcome in patients diagnosed with hand ischemia. *J Vasc Surg* 22:361–369, 1995.
2. Bouhoutos J, Morris T, Martin P: Unilateral Raynaud's phenomenon in the hand and its significance. *Surgery* 82:547, 1977.

3. Janevski BK: Anatomy of the arterial system of the upper extremities, in Janevski B, ed. *Angiography of the Upper Extremity.* The Hague, M Nijhoff, 1982, pp 41–122.
4. Jones NF: Ischemia of the hand in systemic disease. *Clin Plast Surg* 16:547–556, 1989.
5. Thompson JE: Acute peripheral arterial occlusions. *N Engl J Med* 290:950–952, 1974.
6. Coulon M, Goffette P, Dondelinger RF: Local thrombolytic infusion in arterial ischemia of the upper limb: Mid-term results. *Cardiovasc Intervent Radiol* 17:81–86, 1994.
7. Baird RJ, Lajos TZ: Emboli to the arm. *Ann Surg* 160:905, 1964.
8. Conn J Jr, Bergan JJ, Bell JL: Hypothenar hammer syndrome: Post-traumatic digital ischemia. *Surgery* 68:1122–1128, 1970.
9. Von Rosen S: Ein fall von thrombose on der arteria ulnaris nach einwirkung von stumpfen gewalt. *Acta Chir Scand* 73:500–506, 1933.
10. Babu SC, Piccorelli GO, Shah PM, et al: Incidence and results of arterial complications among 16,350 patients undergoing cardiac catheterization. *J Vasc Surg* 10:113–116, 1989.
11. Crossland SG, Neviaser RJ: Complications of radial artery catheterization. *Hand* 9:287–290, 1977.
12. Olin JW, Young JR, Graor RA, et al: The changing clinical spectrum of thrombangitis obliterans (Buerger's disease). *Circulation* 82:3–8, 1990.
13. Jones NF, Imbriglia JE, Steen VD, et al: Surgery for scleroderma of the hand. *J Hand Surg* 12:391, 1987.
14. Mactier RA, Stewart WK, Parham DM, et al: Acral gangrene attributed to calcific azotaemic arteriopathy and the steal effect of an arteriovenous fistula. *Nephron* 54:347–350, 1990.
15. Rubinger D, Friedlaender MM, Silver J, et al: Progressive vascular calcification with necrosis of extremities in hemodialysis patients: A possible role of iron over-load. *Am J Kidney Dis* 7:125–129, 1986.
16. Khatri VP, Gaulin JC, Amin AK: Fibromuscular dysplasia of distal radial and ulnar arteries: Uncommon cause of digital ischemia. *Ann Plast Surg* 33:653–655, 1994.
17. Allen EV, Brown GE: Raynaud's disease: A clinical study of 147 cases. *JAMA* 99:1472, 1932.
18. Priollet T, Vayssairat M, Housset E: How to classify Raynaud's phenomenon. *Am J Med* 83:494–498, 1987.
19. Kahaleh B, Matucci-Cerinic M: Raynaud's phenomenon in scleroderma: Dysregulated neuroendothelial control of vascular tone. *Arthritis Rheum* 38:1–4, 1995.
20. Kallenberg CG: Early detection of connective tissue disease in patients with Raynaud's phenomenon. *Rheum Dis Clin North Am* 16:11–30, 1990.
21. Miller LM, Morgan RF: Vasospastic disorders. *Hand Clin* 9:171–187, 1993.
22. Koman LA, Smith BP, Smith TL: Stress testing in the evaluation of upper extremity perfusion. *Hand Clin* 9:59–83, 1993.

23. Merritt WH: Comprehensive management of Raynaud's syndrome. *Clin Plast Surg* 24:133–159, 1997.

24. Wilgis EFS: Digital sympathectomy for vascular insufficiency. *Hand Clin* 1:361, 1985.

25. Jejurikar SS, Zachary LS: The efficacy of digital sympathectomy with adventitial stripping in scleroderma patients who are "non-responders" to cold stress testing. American Association of Hand Surgery, Abstract, Scientific Paper Session 5 program, p 104, Scottsdale, Ariz, 1998.

26. Bounameaux H, Schneider PA, Huber-Sauteur E, et al: Severe ischemia of the hand following intra-arterial promazine injection: Effects of vasodilation, anticoagulation, and local thrombolysis with tissue-type plasminogen activator. *Vasa* 19:68–71, 1990.

27. Wildus DM, Venbrux AC, Benenati JF, et al: Fibrinolytic therapy for upper-extremity arterial occlusions. [see comments] *Radiology* 175:393–399, 1990.

28. Hirshberg A, Schneiderman J, Garniek A, et al: Errors and pitfalls in intraarterial thrombolytic therapy. *J Vasc Surg* 10:612–616, 1989.

29. Sullivan KL, Minken SL, White RI Jr: Treatment of a case of thromboembolism resulting from thoracic outlet syndrome with intra-arterial urokinase infusion. *J Vasc Surg* 7:568–571, 1988.

30. Yakubov SJ, Nappi JF, Candela RJ, et al: Successful prolonged local infusion of urokinase for the hypothenar hammer syndrome. *Cathet Cardiovasc Diagn* 29:301–303, 1992.

31. Baker RJ, Chunprapaph B, Nyhus LM: Severe ischemia of the hand following radial artery catheterization. *Surgery* 80:449–457, 1976.

32. Koman LA, Smith BP, Pollock FE Jr, et al: The microcirculatory effects of peripheral sympathectomy. *J Hand Surg* 20A:709–717, 1995.

33. eL Gammal TA, Blair WF: Digital periarterial sympathectomy for ischemic digital pain and ulcers. *J Hand Surg [Br]* 16:382–385, 1991.

34. Pederson WC: Management of severe ischemia of the upper extremity. *Clin Plast Surg* 24:107–120, 1997.

35. Silcott GR, Polich VL: Palmar arch arterial reconstruction for the salvage of ischemic fingers. *Am J Surg* 142:219–225, 1981.

36. Barral X, Favre JP, Gournier JP, et al: Late results of palmar arch bypass in the treatment of digital trophic disorders. *Ann Vasc Surg* 6:418–424, 1992.

37. Nehler MR, Dalman RL, Harris EJ, et al: Upper extremity arterial bypass distal to the wrist. *J Vasc Surg* 16:633–640, 1992. [discussion 640–642.]

38. Guzman-Stein G, Schubert W, Najarian DW, et al: Composite in situ vein bypass for upper extremity revascularization. *Plast Reconstr Surg* 83:533–536, 1989.

39. Ristow AV, Cury JM, Costa EL, et al: Revascularization of the ischaemic hand using in situ veins. *Cardiovasc Surg* 4:466–469, 1996.

40. Kniemeyer HW, Sandmann W: In situ and composite in situ vein bypass for upper extremity ischaemia. *Eur J Vasc Surg* 6:41–46, 1992.

41. Baffour R, Danylewick R, Burdon T, et al: An angiographic study of ischemia as a determinant of neovascularization in arteriovenous reversal. *Surg Gynecol Obstet* 166:28–32, 1988.

42. Graham AM, Baffour R, Burdon T, et al: A demonstration of vascular proliferation in response to arteriovenous reversal in the ischemic canine hind limb. *J Surg Res* 47:341–347, 1989.

43. Goldsmith HS: Salvage of end-stage ischemic extremities by intact omentum. *Surgery* 88:732–736, 1980.

44. Herrera HR, Geary J, Whitehead P, et al: Revascularization of the lower extremity with omentum. *Clin Plast Surg* 18:491–495, 1991.

45. Maurya SD, Singhal S, Gupta HC, et al: Pedicled omental grafts in the revascularization of ischemic lower limbs in Buerger's disease. *Int Surg* 70:253–255, 1985.

46. Pederson WC, Pribaz JJ: Revascularization of the upper extremity with microsurgical omental transfer, when faced with end-stage ischemia. *J Reconstr Microsurg* 11:397, 1995.

PART V

Lower Extremity Ischemia

CHAPTER 10

Role of Duplex Imaging Before Infrainguinal Bypass

D.E. Strandness, Jr., M.D.

Professor, Department of Surgery, University of Washington School of Medicine, Seattle, Washington

A fter the first article on the potential role for ultrasonic duplex scanning in 1974, progress in bringing this technology to clinical practice accelerated throughout the 1980s.[1, 2] The method initially was used only for study of the carotid arteries, but as improvements in the technology occurred, duplex scanning was applied to many other areas of the circulation.[3, 4] The major problems that delayed the use of this technology in other anatomical areas were related to the depth of the vessels of interest, combined with the need to verify the accuracy of the method in comparison with angiography.[5] Once all the vessels of interest could be reached with ultrasound, the documentation of its utility was not long in coming.[6–8] However, it was not certain to what extent this relatively new technology would influence clinical practice.

The routine evaluation of patients with peripheral arterial disease has in the past consisted of an appropriate history and physical examination, followed by arteriography if the patient was considered a candidate for some form of intervention. Under these circumstances, it is interesting to speculate how duplex scanning might influence the work-up and therapy of peripheral vascular common problems. It is convenient, for example, to discuss lower extremity arterial disease because it involves specific segments of the arterial system. Atherosclerotic involvement can conveniently be divided into proximal (above the inguinal ligament), mid (common femoral to popliteal), and distal (popliteal to pedal vessels). If revascularization of the limbs is decided upon, the choice of treatment will be entirely dependent on the location and extent of the anatomical lesions. If the disease is confined to the proximal areas of the arterial system, then treatment will be either some form of endovascular therapy or direct arterial surgery, or a combined approach.

Our first efforts using duplex scanning were to determine whether we could identify patients who might be eligible for transluminal angioplasty.[9] If a patient were considered a candidate for intervention of any kind, a duplex scan was done to assess the likelihood that an angioplasty would be of value. If an appropriate lesion were found, the patient was counseled to this end and a request was made to the interventional radiologist to proceed with planning for the procedure. There were 122 patients in this study, with 110 (82%) having their arteriographic studies done after their duplex scans. There were 50 patients who were scheduled for angioplasty on the basis of the findings from the duplex scan. The angioplasty was done in 47 (94%). There were three cases in which the procedure was not performed. In one case, the lesion at the common iliac bifurcation was considered to be too risky to dilate. In the second case, the lesion found on duplex was seen but did not have a measurable pressure gradient. In the third patient, the short stenosis in the proximal superficial femoral artery was associated with a downstream occlusion that had been missed.

Because the majority of our current surgical approaches to chronic limb ischemia are for disease distal to the inguinal ligament, it is legitimate to question how duplex scanning might influence our management. Like many other changes in practice, the use of this technology is still evolving, but one can be confident that duplex scanning will play an increasingly important role in this area. The opinions in this article are based upon experience over a period of many years with this method. There are many constraints on our practice, not the least of which is conservation of resources. If duplex scanning is to play a role, it must neither add to the cost of the current approach nor contribute to the morbidity and mortality rate of the therapeutic procedure.

BYPASS CONDUIT

There is no argument that autologous vein is the desirable bypass material for infrainguinal bypass. It has a proven track record in terms of long-term patency.[10–12] If a vein is to be used for the bypass, it is necessary, of course, to have a vein that is of adequate length and diameter.[13] In general, the greater saphenous vein is the most desirable. To assess its utility, vascular surgeons have to depend upon physical examination or some imaging method to document its availability and suitability. All vascular surgeons have been in the unenviable position of exploring the saphenous vein at the time of surgery, only to find that it is not adequate. This led some to recommend venography as a method of documentation, but venography has not always been satisfactory for some of the following reasons: (1) it is painful and costly; (2) it has to be done bilaterally if the ipsilateral vein is found to be inadequate; and (3) the dimensions seen on the venogram may differ from those found during surgery. In addition, as vascular surgeons gained experience, it became apparent that, if necessary, alternative veins, such as the lesser saphenous or arm veins, could also be used to bypass areas of disease.[14, 15] It was obviously impractical to recommend venograms for assessing all of these alternate sites.

As the technology regarding near-field resolution improved, it became relatively simple to assess the total length of any venous segment and determine its caliber and possible suitability as a bypass conduit. I have had several personal experiences that have convinced me that preoperative scanning and marking is essential:

1. The fruitless search for a suitable vein in both legs without preoperative imaging.
2. The loss of a skin flap when the dissection in the upper thigh was too extensive, which could have been avoided if the exact pathway of the greater saphenous vein had been known and marked on the skin.
3. The finding of large and suitable "greater saphenous" veins that had been presumably used for bypass by other surgeons. This has happened to me on two separate occasions.
4. The finding of dual systems before the procedure itself, making me aware of what to expect.

Although it is difficult to prove whether preliminary venous duplex imaging has made operative procedures more successful or durable, it has become an integral part of our approach to this type of surgical procedure. When we enter the operating room, we know which veins are available, their size, and their length. This has made our task much simpler.

DOCUMENTATION OF SITES OF DISEASE

Irrespective of the potential role for any new imaging procedure, there already is a great deal of historical information concerning the anatomical distribution of lower extremity arterial disease and its impact on limb function and survival. Although it is always dangerous to generalize, we do know the following[16-19]:

1. Claudication of moderate severity is usually associated with a single level of occlusion or stenosis.
2. When the claudication becomes incapacitating, it is generally caused by multilevel disease.
3. Type 2 diabetics have a different distribution of disease, which can be summarized as follows[16, 17, 19]:

- They have a lower incidence of aortoiliac disease.
- There is a similar incidence of femoropopliteal disease.
- There is a much higher incidence of tibial-peroneal involvement.
- Medial calcification is found in the tibial and peroneal arteries of the diabetic. This can easily be detected by duplex scanning.
- The type 2 diabetic has a very high incidence of peripheral neuropathy.[19]

Given these historical facts, it is possible to know at the outset what might be expected when the patient is first evaluated. Of course the physical examination will help in localization of the disease, but it lacks precision.[20]

STRATEGY FOR THERAPY

As noted above, the clinical presentation will guide us in fairly accurate terms as to what might be needed if an intervention is required or sought by the patient. For mild to moderately severe claudication, the disease that is responsible may involve only a single segment, which makes the decision-making process quite simple. For example, if the patient has calf, thigh, and hip pain with exercise, together with palpable foot pulses and an associated bruit heard in the iliac artery area, the diagnosis of common iliac stenosis is very likely and transluminal angioplasty with or without a stent probably is the treatment of choice.[21, 22] On the other hand, anything beyond this in terms of severity of symptoms or absence of pulses makes predictions more difficult and requires more information. For the patient with critical ischemia, multisegment disease is nearly always the rule and may require more than one therapeutic effort to take care of the problem. In my therapeutic approach to patients, I place them in one of the following disease categories:

1. Proximal aortoiliac disease with superficial femoral involvement, but a patent popliteal artery and one or more patent runoff vessels.
2. Proximal disease with superficial femoral–popliteal artery occlusion and one or more patent runoff vessels.
3. No proximal disease, but stenoses or occlusions confined to the superficial femoral artery with a patent popliteal artery.
4. No proximal disease, but an occluded superficial femoral–popliteal artery with one or more patent runoff vessels.
5. No proximal disease, but an occluded superficial femoral–popliteal segment with patent vessels at the level of the distal leg and foot.

Each of these scenarios requires imaging of one type or another to define the location and extent of the arterial occlusive disease. If arteriography is considered alone, the instances in which adequate visualization is or can be a problem are seen with patients in categories 4 and 5. This has led to alternative methods of study, such as inflow occlusion during injection of the dye or the use of magnetic resonance arteriography (MRA) for visualization of the arteries in the distal limb. With the exception of the patient having isolated disease in the aortoiliac area, any therapeutic approach often will require some form of proximal intervention in conjunction with a distal procedure. The proximal procedure will consist of either some endovascular procedure or a direct surgical approach (aortofemoral or cross-femoral grafting procedure).

ROLE OF DUPLEX SCANNING

The role of duplex scanning will depend entirely on the questions asked and the kind of information that needs to be obtained. This will influence the nature of the study itself, the type of data obtained, the algorithm that is chosen to be used, and its accuracy compared with standard arteriographic procedures/intra-arterial pressure measurements. At the outset, it is important to point out that the variability of arteriographic assessment even using calipers is very large. The problem is compounded further by the lack of multiple views.[6, 23–26] My experience with duplex scanning of peripheral arteries was divided into two phases. The first was to establish some criteria for the detection of hemodynamically significant stenoses. In practice, a hemodynamically significant stenosis is one that produces an abnormal pressure gradient. This is generally caused by a lesion that reduces lumen diameter by greater than 50%.[21] However, some lesions that reduce diameter by less may produce a gradient that is significant when flow is increased to meet the needs of the exercising muscle.[22, 27]

Normally, the peak systolic velocity (PSV) in the arterial tree will gradually decrease as one proceeds from the level of the abdominal aorta to the pedal arteries. In the aorta, the PSV will be in the range of 100 cm/sec with a standard deviation of ± 20%. It is this wide standard deviation that makes it difficult to use absolute velocity values for the classification of the degree of narrowing. However, there is one feature of the arterial velocity patterns that remains very constant in normal subjects, and that is the triphasic flow pattern (forward-reverse-forward flow). This feature will be preserved to the level of the ankle and is a good marker. For example, if a triphasic flow pattern is observed in the common femoral artery, it is very unlikely that there is a significant lesion proximal to that level. Although I have observed restoration of a triphasic flow pattern distal to a high-grade stenosis, it is very uncommon.[28, 29]

It is important to realize that, even with the development of high-resolution scanners, it is impossible to use the image of a lesion alone to determine its hemodynamic severity. There is no doubt that lesions can be seen and the presence of medial calcification in tibial-peroneal vessels can be determined, but it is impossible to grade lesions merely by their appearance. One must depend upon the hemodynamic changes that are observed across suspected areas of disease. To accomplish this task, it is necessary to follow certain rules. Some of these are as follows:

1. The entire length of the arterial supply should be scanned. There is a perception that scanning of the aortoiliac segments cannot be done, but this is not true. Patients should be studied in the fasting state to minimize bowel gas, which will help a great deal.
2. The pulsed Doppler sample volume is swept through the length of the arterial segment to document any sudden changes in the PSV. The criteria for grading a stenosis are as follows:

• Normally, there should be no increase in PSV from one segment to another.
• If there is an increase in the PSV from one segment to another, and it is less than 100%, and there is preservation of reverse flow, the lesion reduces diameter by less than 50%.

- If the PSV increases by more than 100% from one point to the next, the stenosis is greater than 50%.
- With occlusions, there is no detectable flow.[5, 6]

Most laboratories express the data in terms of PSV at the site of the stenosis divided by that found immediately proximal to that area. A ratio above 1.5 in my study, and slightly higher (greater than 2.0) from other studies, is taken as representing hemodynamically significant disease.[26]

What about the use of color duplex alone? Hatsukami et al.[28, 30] used color duplex in comparison with arteriography to determine its use for the detection of hemodynamically significant stenoses and total occlusions. The criteria used were as follows:

1. A triphasic color shift was labeled as normal.
2. Poststenotic turbulence, which is seen as an admixture of colors, was interpreted as being consistent with a hemodynamically significant stenosis.
3. Absence of detectable flow with the visualization of collaterals was assumed to reflect a total occlusion.

The conclusions of the study were that color duplex alone could be used for broad classification of disease, but that it should not be used in isolation or as the sole method of study.

As noted in the study by Jager et al.,[5] when the results of duplex scanning are compared with arteriography and the readings of one radiologist compared with another, scanning performs very well (Tables 1 and 2). In fact, it is this observation that suggests it may be possible to use this noninvasive modality as a method of selecting the appropriate operative procedure. To test this feasibility, Kohler et al.[7] took the anatomical information obtained from arteriography and duplex scanning to construct a chart of the circulation. The other data provided were the reason for the study, the ankle/arm index, and the results of a treadmill test if it had been done. This information was sent to six vascular surgeons, who were asked to indicate the procedure they would use given the data sent to them. They did not know whether the information provided was from the duplex scan or the arteriogram. They were given the following options: (1) no intervention; (2) percutaneous angioplasty; (3) operative endarterectomy; (4) aortobifemoral bypass; (5) femorofemoral bypass; (6) femoropopliteal bypass; (7) combined aortofemoral bypass and femoropopliteal bypass; and (8) other options.

The studies from 29 patients were included in the material that was sent to the six participating surgeons. The intraobserver agree-

TABLE 1.

Comparison of Duplex Scanning and Arteriography (< 50% vs. > 50%)*

Arterial Segment	Sensitivity (%)	Specificity (%)	Positive Predictive Value (%)	Negative Predictive Value (%)
Iliac	81	100	100	92
Common femoral	56	96	71	91
Superficial femoral—proximal	71	100	100	98
Superficial femoral—mid	80	100	100	88
Superficial femoral—distal	77	90	77	90
Popliteal	80	100	100	93
All segments	77	98	94	92

*There were 30 patients studied.
(Courtesy of Jager KA, Phillips DJ, Martin RL, et al: Noninvasive mapping of lower limb arterial lesions. *Ultrasound Med Biol* 11:515–521. Copyright 1985 by World Federation of Ultrasound in Medicine and Biology. Reprinted by permission of Elsevier Science, Inc.)

ment between surgeons was good (mean Kappa 0.70), with exact agreement in 76% of the cases. The interobserver agreement was less favorable (mean Kappa 0.56). There was significant disagreement in 43% of the cases in which the data from the duplex study and arteriogram were identical. This suggested that the differences were in the decision-making process and not on the basis of the presented data. This should not be too surprising, given the types of discussions that take place during a vascular conference. For example, for unilateral iliac artery disease, one surgeon might prefer a unilateral aortofemoral graft, whereas another, a cross-femoral graft. The same often applies to infrainguinal bypass, depending upon the site and extent of disease. Therefore, the utility of duplex scanning alone often will be determined by the information that any single surgeon might require before proceeding with an operative procedure. In this regard, it is important to outline some of the potential differences as well as areas where surgeons would generally agree. For this discussion, I will assume that the arterial inflow is normal either by duplex scanning or restoration of normal hemodynamics by either an endovascular procedure or direct arterial surgery.

TABLE 2.
Comparison of Angiographer 1 vs. Angiographer 2 ($<$ 50% vs. $>$ 50%)*

Arterial Segment	Sensitivity (%)	Specificity (%)	Positive Predictive Value (%)	Negative Predictive Value (%)
Iliac	94	96	94	96
Common femoral	66	100	100	91
Profunda	33	91	40	88
Superficial femoral—proximal	95	100	100	93
Superficial femoral—mid	100	84	82	100
Superficial femoral—distal	91	85	78	94
Popliteal	91	100	100	95
All segments	87	94	88	93

*There were 30 patients studied. The senior radiologist was considered to be the "gold standard" against which a colleague was compared. All calculations were based upon this premise.
(Courtesy of Jager KA, Phillips DJ, Martin RL, et al: Noninvasive mapping of lower limb arterial lesions. *Ultrasound Med Biol* 11:515–521. Copyright 1985 by World Federation of Ultrasound in Medicine and Biology. Reprinted by permission of Elsevier Science, Inc.)

1. For a short segment occlusion of the superficial femoral artery, the bypass that will be used may be in dispute but all would agree that bypassing that area will restore hemodynamics to normal. However, there may be disagreement regarding whether the bypass should be done to the distal superficial femoral artery or to the popliteal artery. The disagreement relates to the nature of the artery itself and the likelihood that the popliteal artery is less diseased and may well be a better target for the distal anastomosis. Imaging studies could be of assistance in this case if they showed that there was disease in the distal superficial femoral artery, even though it was not hemodynamically significant. Certainly, arteriography might provide this information, but what about duplex scanning? There is no doubt that ultrasound can detect the presence of calcification and provide some information about arterial wall pathology, but its use for this specific purpose has not yet been defined. If it is assumed that either surgical approach is used and is hemodynamically successful initially, then the only ar-

gument would be over its long-term outcome. This has not been determined.

2. If the popliteal trifurcation is occluded, the issues that remain are with respect to the runoff arteries. The concerns in this case are as follows:

- How many are patent?
- How big are the vessels?
- Over what length are they patent?
- Do they communicate with the foot?
- Are the vessels calcified?

With regard to the runoff arteries, the discussion in the past was often related to single-, double-, or triple-vessel runoff and its relationship to long-term patency. This debate has subsided because we now know that a single-vessel runoff is compatible with good long-term results, and that an operation should not be denied on this basis alone. The length of runoff arteries is also irrelevant because we now appreciate that long bypasses, even to the level of the foot, can be done with good long-term outcome. The diameter of the outflow arteries is also important, but no one to my knowledge has been able to relate long-term outcome to this particular variable. It is clear to me that vessels with an inside diameter of 1.5–2.0 mm can be used as an outflow artery for either an in situ or reversed saphenous vein graft. Do the arteries communicate with the foot? This is obviously important, but pathologic studies have in general showed that atherosclerosis (in the absence of renal failure) does not usually affect the vessels of the foot. Although it had been thought that this was not true in the type 2 diabetic, this assumption has been shown to be inaccurate. Calcification of distal arteries comes in two forms: that associated with atherosclerosis vs. that associated with diabetes mellitus. The calcification seen with diabetes is in the media and bears no relationship to that observed with the complicated plaque. Whereas medial calcification was once thought to be a contraindication to the use of such an artery for bypass, this is no longer the case.

Arteriography will often provide nearly all the above information to the satisfaction of the surgeon. However, with extensive arterial disease, flow may not be sufficient to the level of the distal limb to be seen by arteriography. What then? Some surgeons have simply cutdown on the artery with the guidance of Doppler interrogation and then performed an operative arteriogram. There has been some interest in MRA for this purpose, but I do not believe there is enough experience to document its cost-effectiveness. What about duplex? It unquestionably can provide similar information, as shown by the studies of Hatsukami et al.[28, 30]

DISCUSSION

It seems to this observer that we are in a transition phase with regard to the application of duplex scanning as a major contributor or definitive study before infrainguinal bypass. Even considering this as a possible imaging technique to be used alone is a revolutionary concept. The use of arteriography is so ingrained in the minds of physicians that it is going to be very difficult to change their established attitudes. Nevertheless, many other changes have occurred in my professional lifetime, and they have been just as dramatic. For example, who would have ever considered doing a carotid endarterectomy without the performance of an arteriogram of the aortic arch, the carotid bifurcation, the siphon, and the intracranial vessels? Yet, there is a move in this direction that I do not believe can be stopped, given the cost savings, reduction of risk, and evidence that the outcome of intervention is not materially influenced by this change.[31-34] At first glance, this approach seems inappropriate because it encourages an operation based on limited information. However, the notion that carotid endarterectomy could be recommended with only "limited" information came about when intravenous digital subtraction arteriography was introduced as the ideal method for outpatient study, despite the fact that it provided less-than-optimal pictures of the bulb, and very inadequate views of the arch and intracranial vessels. Nevertheless, during the era in which operations were done on the basis of this test alone, the outcome did not appear to be any different. Also, the results of the Asymptomatic Carotid Endarterectomy Trial clearly showed that the stroke rate with arteriography was nearly equal to that seen with operation.[35] In addition, the cost savings in avoiding the contrast study are very significant even without factoring in the cost of its complications.

The situation with regard to the legs is, in some respects, simpler, but in other respects, more complicated. In the legs, we are interested in identifying those segments of the circulation that have lesions reducing pressure and flow to the limb. As already discussed, this involves identifying these lesions and then properly planning the operative procedure. For lesions proximal to the inguinal ligament, we are, in a sense, in competition with the endovascular therapist who must have an arteriogram to complete the task at hand. However, there is convincing evidence that we can be of assistance in determining who may need the procedure and which site of access is most likely to lead to a satisfactory outcome.

Below the inguinal ligament, the problems are a bit different in the sense that endovascular procedures are not as durable as one might like, and they cannot be used for many of the very extensive lesions that we see and I am asked to treat. Assuming duplex could provide the same kind of information that arteriography does during evaluation, then there is no reason why it could not be used as the primary method for determining the course of intervention. Taking this stand, I would like to provide the following scenario in which this might be appropriate:

1. Documentation of lesions in the external iliac and common femoral areas is not a problem.
2. The profunda femoris artery is accessible.
3. The superficial femoral artery can be easily examined throughout its length.
4. The proximal popliteal artery and its course through the fossa can be accessed with little trouble.
5. The bifurcation of the posterior tibial and the peroneal arteries can be seen.
6. The origin of the anterior tibial artery is not difficult to see.
7. The tibial vessels can be followed throughout their length.

What, then, are the problems? At the moment, the most difficult situation for duplex scanning is with multilevel disease that is associated with very low flow in the tibial and peroneal arteries. What does very low flow mean from an anatomical and disease standpoint? Although it is possible to detect very low velocities (less than 10 cm/sec), at what point can one say that a peripheral artery is not suitable for placing the distal anastomosis of a graft? Presently, there is no answer to this very important question, and it will not be answered until a carefully controlled case study is done.

In the interim, is there a satisfactory compromise until such data are accumulated? I believe so, and would suggest the following:

1. For an occlusion confined to the superficial femoral artery, an arteriogram is not necessary. The arteriogram would only confirm what we already know. Some surgeons prefer to use the popliteal artery as the distal site for graft implantation, but this

choice is determined by the empirical view that the popliteal artery is less likely to have disease involvement than the distal superficial femoral artery. It should also be noted that with high-resolution ultrasound, it is becoming easier to identify wall changes in arteries of this size.

2. If there is an occlusion that involves the popliteal artery and the trifurcation, but there is three-vessel runoff by duplex, then surgeons could pick their artery of choice for bypass. What artery should be chosen? Perhaps this could be based upon the velocity information or, again, surgical preference. For example, it is known that the peroneal artery is less likely to be involved than the other two tibial arteries and can serve as an excellent outflow vessel. My own preference in this situation would be to use the peroneal artery.

3. If there is two-vessel runoff with good flow by duplex in both, again the procedure could be that which is most comfortable for the surgeon. For example, if the surgeon is prone to use in situ grafting, this could influence the site of implantation.

4. If the flow velocity is very low (less than 20 cm/sec) in one or more of the distal vessels, this would provide the greatest dilemma. This is also the situation in which arteriography will often have problems as well. It may well be that this decision could be best made at the time of operation with an operative arteriogram.

This approach has been applied on only a limited scale, but it is clear to me that it represents the trend of the future. I see no evidence to date that it will provide a poorer outcome. It is important that we not become dogmatic in an area undergoing dynamic changes. For example, at one time it was not considered feasible or useful to extend bypass grafts to the distal leg. This was wrong. It was also thought by some that diabetics could not profit by distal bypasses because of microvascular disease in the foot. This was wrong.[18] Some felt that calcification of tibial vessels precluded successful grafting. This was wrong.

Finally, we have been forced to economize on the delivery of care without sacrificing outcome. This has been frustrating, but at the same time has forced us to rethink why we do what we do, and how we can change. It is my view that the use of duplex scanning in the selection of patients for lower extremity revascularization is an area where vascular surgeons can have a big impact on the cost of health care in this country.

REFERENCES

1. Barber FE, Baker DW, Nation AWC, et al: Ultrasonic duplex echo Doppler scanner. *IEEE Trans Biomed Eng* 21:109–113, 1974.
2. Barber FE, Baker DW, Strandness DE Jr: Duplex scanner II for simultaneous imaging of artery tissues and flow. *Ultrasonics Symposium Proc IEEE* 74CH0896-ISU, 1974.
3. Blackshear WM, Phillips DJ, Thiele BL, et al: Detection of carotid occlusive disease by ultrasonic imaging and pulsed Doppler spectral analysis. *Surgery* 86:698, 1979.
4. Phillips DJ, Powers JE, Eyer MK, et al: Detection of peripheral vascular disease using duplex scanner III. *Ultrasound Med Biol* 6:205–218, 1980.
5. Jager KA, Phillips DJ, Martin RL, et al: Noninvasive mapping of lower limb arterial lesions. *Ultrasound Med Biol* 11:515–521, 1985.
6. Kohler TR, Nance DR, Cramer MM, et al: Duplex scanning for diagnosis of aortoiliac and femoropopliteal disease: A prospective study. *Circulation* 76:1074–1080, 1987.
7. Kohler TR, Andros G, Porter JM, et al: Can duplex scanning replace arteriography for lower extremity arterial disease? *Ann Vasc Surg* 4:280–287, 1990.
8. Cossman DV, Ellison JE, Wagner WH, et al: Comparison of contrast arteriography to arterial mapping with color-flow imaging in the lower extremities. *J Vasc Surg* 10:522–529, 1989.
9. Edwards JM, Coldwell DM, Goldman ML, et al: The role of duplex scanning in the selection of patients for transluminal angioplasty. *J Vasc Surg* 13:69–74, 1991.
10. Bandyk DF, Schmitt DD, Seabrook GR, et al: Monitoring functional patency of in situ saphenous vein bypasses: The impact of a surveillance protocol and elective revision. *J Vasc Surg* 9:286–296, 1989.
11. Bandyk DF: Postoperative surveillance of infrainguinal bypass. *Surg Clin North Am* 70:71–75, 1990.
12. Mills JL, Bandyk DF, Gahtan V, et al: The origin of infrainguinal vein graft stenosis: A prospective study based on duplex surveillance. *J Vasc Surg* 21:16–22, 1995.
13. Leather RP, Kupinski AM: Preoperative evaluation of the saphenous vein as a suitable graft. *Semin Vasc Surg* 1:51, 1988.
14. Salles-Cunha SX, Beebe HG, Andros G: Preoperative assessment of alternative veins. *Semin Vasc Surg* 8:172–178, 1995.
15. Apyan RL, Schneider PA, Andros G: Preservation of arm veins for arterial reconstruction. *J Vasc Nurs* 10:2–5, 1992.
16. Wheelock FC Jr: Transmetatarsal amputation and arterial surgery in diabetic patients. *N Engl J Med* 264:316–320, 1961.
17. Gensler SW, Haimovici H, Hoffert P, et al: Study of vascular lesions in diabetic, non-diabetic patients. *Arch Surg* 91:617–622, 1965.
18. Rosenblum BI, Pomposelli FB Jr, Giurini JM, et al: Maximizing foot salvage by a combined approach to foot ischemia and neuropathic ul-

ceration in patients with diabetes: A 5-year experience. *Diabetes Care* 17:983–987, 1994.

19. Strandness DE Jr, Priest RR, Gibbons GE: A combined clinical and pathological study of nondiabetic and diabetic vascular disease. *Diabetes* 13:366–372, 1964.

20. Marinelli MR, Beach KW, Glass MJ, et al: Noninvasive testing vs. clinical evaluation of arterial disease: A prospective study. *JAMA* 241:2031–2034, 1979.

21. May AG, Vandeberg L, DeWeese JA, et al: Critical arterial stenosis. *Surgery* 54:250–259, 1963.

22. Carter SA: Response of ankle systolic pressure to leg exercise in mild or questionable arterial disease. *N Engl J Med* 287:578–582, 1972.

23. Jager KA: Measurement of mesenteric blood flow by duplex scanning. *J Vasc Surg* 3:462–469, 1986.

24. Thiele BL, Strandness DE Jr: Accuracy of angiographic quantification of peripheral atherosclerosis. *Prog Cardiovasc Dis* 26:223–236, 1983.

25. Elsman BH, Legemate DA, van-der-Heyden FW, et al: The use of color-coded duplex scanning in the selection of patients with lower-extremity arterial disease for percutaneous transluminal angioplasty: A prospective study. *Cardiovasc Intervent Radiol* 19:313–316, 1996.

26. Elsman BH, Legemate DA, van-der-Heijden FH, et al: Impact of ultrasonographic duplex scanning on therapeutic decision-making in lower-limb arterial disease. *Br J Surg* 82:630–633, 1995.

27. Carter SA: Arterial auscultation in peripheral vascular disease. *JAMA* 246:1682–1686, 1981.

28. Hatsukami TS, Primozich JP, Zierler RE, et al: Color Doppler imaging of lower-extremity arterial disease: A prospective validation study. *J Vasc Surg* 16:527–533, 1992.

29. Strandness DE Jr: *Duplex Scanning in Vascular Disorders,* ed 2. New York, Raven Press, 1993.

30. Hatsukami TS, Primozich J, Zierler RE, et al: Color Doppler characteristics in normal lower-extremity arteries. *Ultrasound Med Biol* 16: 167–171, 1992.

31. Dawson DL, Zierler RE, Kohler TR: Role of arteriography in the preoperative evaluation of carotid artery disease. *Am J Surg* 161:619–624, 1991.

32. Dawson DL, Zierler RE, Strandness DE Jr, et al: The role of duplex scanning and arteriography before carotid endarterectomy: A prospective study. *J Vasc Surg* 18:673–683, 1993.

33. Moore WS, Ziomek S, Quinones-Baldrich WJ, et al: Can clinical evaluation and noninvasive testing substitute for arteriography in the evaluation of carotid artery disease? *Ann Surg* 208:91–94, 1988.

34. Ricotta JJ, Holen J, Schenk E, et al: Is routine arteriography necessary prior to carotid endarterectomy? *J Vasc Surg* 1:96–102, 1984.

35. Executive Committee Asymptomatic Carotid Atherosclerosis Study: Endarterectomy for asymptomatic carotid artery stenosis. *JAMA* 273:1421–1428, 1995.

CHAPTER 11

Role of Magnetic Resonance Angiography in Peripheral Vascular Disease

William D. Turnipseed, M.D.
Professor, Department of Surgery, Section of Vascular Surgery, University of Wisconsin Hospital and Clinics, Madison, Wisconsin

Thomas M. Grist, M.D.
Associate Professor, Department of Radiology, University of Wisconsin Hospital and Clinics, Madison, Wisconsin

The traditional use of contrast arteriography in the preoperative evaluation of patients with symptoms of cerebrovascular and peripheral ischemia has changed as less invasive methods of arterial imaging have become available. The fact that traditional contrast X-ray arteriography is costly, interventional, and not completely safe (stroke and death rate, 0.1% to 1%; catheter-induced hemorrhage, 2%; embolization, 2%) has encouraged development of techniques such as noninvasive magnetic resonance angiography (MRA). Magnetic resonance imaging (MRI) utilizes an electromagnetic field to create differential atomic signals in soft tissues. This is a multifaceted, noninvasive diagnostic technique that makes it possible to evaluate the structural anatomy of the arterial circulation and to acquire functional information about arterial blood flow without interventional catheterization or intra-arterial injection of contrast agents. A variety of MRI techniques have been devised to provide arterial imaging based on functional blood flow patterns and velocities. Arterial image acquisition is most commonly achieved using time-of-flight (TOF) or phase contrast (PC) pulse sequences.

Two-dimensional (2D) TOF is the most commonly used technique in the evaluation of the peripheral vascular circulation. This is a gradient-recalled echo technique, which uses radio frequency pulses to suppress signals from surrounding soft tissue, and is based on the concept that blood flowing into a given field of view (high signal) appears bright in relationship to adjacent saturated soft tissues (low signal). In TOF arteriography, thin cross-sections of soft tissue are saturated by radio frequency pulses. Blood that is outside the slice volume (1.5-mm thick) is fully relaxed and magnetized, and as it enters the slice volume, it appears bright compared with the surrounding saturated soft tissues. The best vascular images result from rapid entry and exit of blood through the saturated soft tissue volume and occur because of a phenomenon known as "flow-related enhancement." When blood transit through the saturated soft tissue slice is slow, it will be pulsed many times as it passes through the slice, and it will lose signal intensity. Two-dimensional TOF uses small flip angles and short repetition times that provide rapid imaging sequences without significant degradation of signal-to-noise ratios. The advantages of 2D TOF angiography include minimum saturation effects for normal flow velocities, short acquisition time, and increased sensitivity to the presence of low-flow states in the circulation. This method of arterial imaging has been most commonly used in the clinical assessment of the cervical carotid arteries and/or imaging of the distal runoff vessels in the lower extremity and feet. Major disadvantages of TOF include sensitivity to flow traveling in the same plane as the imaging slice, motion-related artifacts, and a tendency to overestimate the severity of stenosis.

An alternative form of TOF imaging is three-dimensional (3D) acquisition in which much thicker tissue volume slabs are used (3–8 cm in thickness vs. 1.5 mm for 2D TOF). Three-dimensional TOF makes it possible to increase spatial resolution because very thin partitions may be reconstructed (<1-mm thickness) from these volume slabs. Consequently, 3D TOF requires higher blood flow rates but is much less sensitive to intravoxel dephasing caused by turbulent blood flow. For this reason, it is well adapted for the evaluation of the intracranial circulation and the carotid bifurcation. The combination of 2D and 3D TOF imaging allows for the detection of slow flow and also improves spatial resolution. The combined use of these two TOF imaging techniques in a sequential, multiple overlapping thin-slab acquisition (MOTSA), allows for very little saturation of blood as it traverses the slab, thus resulting in high contrast and high resolution images over a large field of view. This combination of techniques has been helpful in resolving some of the major disadvantages associated with TOF, including insensitivity to in-plane flow, motion-related artifacts, and overestimation of stenosis.

Another image acquisition technique used in MRA is referred to as phase contrast angiography (PCA). Image signal intensity in PCA is ultimately proportional to blood flow velocity. The PCA sequences are programmed to assign a specific MR signal phase to each velocity of blood flow. Faster moving protons in blood accumulate greater phase shifts relative to slowly flowing blood. An important factor that distinguishes PCA from other methods is that pixel intensity represents phases or differences in phases, rather than the more familiar size of tissue magnetization. Phase contrast angiography flow encoding results from the application of bipolar magnetic field gradients. Magnetic field gradients can be applied in any direction across the body. Phase contrast angiography relies on the physical principle that spins moving in the direction of a bipolar magnetic field gradient will acquire a phase shift proportional to their velocity and to gradient amplitude and duration.

Phase contrast angiography is often performed in addition to TOF imaging to confirm the presence of stenotic lesions in areas of complex geometric flow and to determine flow velocity data. Advantages of 2D PCA include a sensitivity to fast or slow flow, based on varied velocity encoding, short scan times, and better documentation of vessel morphology with less sensitivity to complex flow pattern artifacts. Disadvantages include an increased sensitivity to signal loss in regions of complex flow, and the fact that single projections are required for each acquisition. Phase contrast angiography can be acquired using 3D volume acquisitions, similar to a 3D TOF gradient-recalled echo volume scan. One advantage of 3D PCA is that acquisition is obtained with very small voxels, thus decreasing the amount of intravoxel dephasing and improving the delineation of complex and turbulent flow. Another advantage is that the volume of imaged data obtained and the vascular structures within the 3D volume can be retrospectively processed and projected into any desired plane. This allows for obtaining oblique views of aneurysms and arteriovenous malformations, and adds tremendous versatility to the analysis of angiographic data. Furthermore, 3D PCA images can be used to create directional flow images. These flow images can be projected in any desired orientation and are obtained throughout the cardiac cycle, so that the signal is proportional to average values. The combined use of TOF and PCA creates the potential for obtaining physiologic and anatomical information about the peripheral circulatory system that exceeds the capacity of contrast arteriography.[1]

The obvious advantages of MRA are its safety and cost efficiency when compared with contrast arteriography. At our institution, the charges for an MRA study are nearly $800 less than for a contrast arteriogram. Like other noninvasive techniques, MRA is safe, because it avoids arterial catheterization. It does not require exposure to radiation, nor does it require use of high-volume ionic contrast agents, which may complicate or threaten renal function. Magnetic resonance angiography has advantages over technology such as duplex ultrasound because it can provide functional and anatomical information about the entire peripheral vascular system. Duplex ultrasonography is limited to evaluation of isolated segments of the intracranial, cervical, thoracoabdominal, and lower extremity circulation, in part because it is very operator dependent and in part because of technical limitations. These technical limitations include depth of focus, the presence of overlapping and tortuous collaterals, and the fact that bony structures limit imaging access and insonation angles, which are essential for accurate determination of flow velocity data.

Unfortunately, MRA is not well suited for use in all patients. It is contraindicated in individuals with cardiac pacers or ferromagnetic surgical clips in the required field of view. To obtain good quality vascular imaging with MRA, appropriate patient screening is required. The best patients are those who are cooperative, able to follow instructions, non-claustrophobic, and in no respiratory distress. Proper patient selection, however, does not guarantee good quality vascular imaging. Magnetic resonance imaging is adversely affected by movement during radio frequency pulse sequences. Swallowing, breathing, intestinal peristalsis, and incidental physical movements can severely degrade image quality. Furthermore, there is a tendency for 2D TOF arteriography to overestimate the severity of stenosis or to incorrectly suggest the presence of occlusive disease, because of turbulent arterial flow or changes in the planar position of the artery relative to the plane of the radio frequency pulse in the magnetic field. "Flow void" or signal loss associated with turbulent flow across hemodynamically significant lesions is a result of complex, turbulent flow causing intravoxel dephasing and loss of signal intensity. These flow artifacts commonly result in overgrading the severity of stenosis. In-plane flow artifacts suggesting occlusion or stenosis can also result from changes in the orientation of blood vessels that occur in areas of complex arterial flow, such as the intracranial and pelvic circulation, or in tortuous collateral circulatory beds. When blood flows in parallel to the saturation plane of a magnetic field during 2D TOF MRA, the resulting signal loss suggests the presence of stenotic or occlusive disease. The presence of metallic clips adjacent to vascular structures, and retrograde flow through collateralized vascular segments in the field of view of a saturation band, may cause patent vascular segments to appear completely occluded. The use of shorter repetition and echo times, elimination of ferromagnetic clips, and PC imaging have helped us significantly reduce these imaging artifact problems.[1, 2]

The recent use of 3D TOF image acquisition, in conjunction with intravenous injection of paramagnetic contrast agents has significantly improved the accuracy and clinical utility of MRA (Fig 1). Three-dimensional TOF uses a T_1-weighted fast gradient echo scan that uses very short echo and repetition times and large flip angles to reduce background signal intensity. Digital subtraction of source images enables processing very similar to digital arteriography. The most commonly used paramagnetic contrast agent is gadolinium. Gadolinium is a heavy metal analogue that is chelated with diethylenetriamine pentaacetic acid (DTPA). This is a potent T_1 relaxing agent in blood and improves arterial imaging because of the increased contrast between blood and surrounding soft tissue. This agent is not nephrotoxic, is excreted by glomerular filtration, and can be used in conjunction with PC imaging to determine glomerular function. Gadolinium (concentration 0.3 mmol/kg) is infused intravenously at a rate of 1.5–2 mL/sec over a 30-second injection. A dose-timing curve is determined so that proper timing of arterial scanning can be calculated for the arterial bed that is to be examined (Fig 2). The combined use of 3D TOF and gadolinium contrast agents has resulted in significant reduction in flow void artifacts, elimination of in-plane flow defects, reduction in imaging time, and improvement in spatial resolution. When these improved arterial imaging techniques are used, overall accuracy compared with traditional contrast arteriography ranges from 92% to 98%, depending on the field of view interrogated. Sensitivity ranges from 83% to 97%, and specificity from 92% to 98%.[3]

One of the major issues regarding contemporary use of MRA has to do with whether it can be used as a sole diagnostic test and effectively eliminate the use of contrast arteriography and noninvasive testing. Unfortunately, there still exists a significant technology gap between centers of research and development and the general medical community, particularly when it comes to image

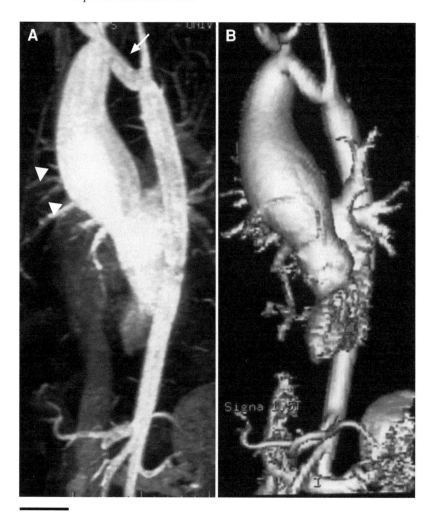

FIGURE 1

Contrast-enhanced MRA of patient with aortic coarctation and ascending aortic aneurysm. **A,** maximum intensity projection (MIP) of the aorta, lateral view demonstrating the aortic coarctation *(arrow)* and the ascending aortic aneurysm *(arrowheads)*. The image represents a MIP display through the entire set of 44 images acquired using a three-dimensional contrast-enhanced gradient echo acquisition. The image was acquired during a 30-second breath-hold. Forty mL of gadodiamide contrast was infused at 2 mL/sec during the acquisition of the images. Note the large field of view and excellent anatomical coverage associated with the technique. **B,** shaded-surfaced display (SSD) of the same data. The SSD provides some additional information regarding the three-dimensional features of the anatomy. In contrast to CT angiography, the bony anatomy is not visualized using the technique, and therefore little additional processing of the images is necessary to eliminate the bony structures.

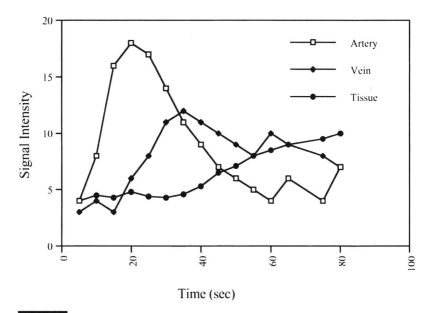

FIGURE 2

Timing diagram for contrast-enhanced MRA. Typical curves for signal intensity vs. time are shown for the arterial system, venous anatomy, and stationary tissues. For arterial phase contrast-enhanced MRA, it is necessary to time the acquisition of the 3-dimensional volume to the arrival of contrast in the arterial vascular bed being evaluated. Appropriate timing causes preferential arterial enhancement relative to the venous phase or stationary tissue phase of contrast passage. Typically, the duration of the acquisition of the contrast-enhanced MRA technique is 30 seconds. In the future, it is likely that shorter duration acquisitions will become available, and therefore multiple time-resolved images will be obtained during the first passage of contrast, similar to digital subtraction techniques used for conventional angiography.

processing. Uniform image processing software packages have not been agreed upon, and paramagnetic contrast agents remain expensive and are not yet widely used. This means that in most centers, 2D and 3D TOF imaging remains the technique for peripheral arteriography. Because there is a high association with image artifacts, confirmatory noninvasive tests are still frequently required, and in many cases contrast arteriography must be performed to resolve artifacts.

CAROTID VASCULATURE

The one clinical area where MRA has resulted in dramatic reduction in the use of contrast arteriography is in the diagnosis and management of cerebrovascular disease. Magnetic resonance angiography has demonstrated the capacity to accurately identify complete arterial occlusion and to distinguish occlusions from severe stenoses with an overall accuracy that exceeds 95%. Sensitivity and specificity for detection of high-grade lesions are 100% and 93%, respectively, at our institution.[4] The capacity of MRA to confirm duplex findings in symptomatic patients has made it possible to avoid costs and additional risk exposure associated with routine preoperative contrast arteriography.[5] Although some would suggest that preoperative duplex imaging is accurate and effective for identifying the presence of hemodynamically significant carotid occlusive disease, this practice is particularly bothersome when it comes to dealing with asymptomatic patients. Duplex imaging is very operator dependent, and accuracy rates vary tremendously from laboratory to laboratory. The practice of basing management decisions on such a test would require that the laboratories be certified by a central accrediting agency, and that diagnostic accuracy and continuing quality assurance surveillance be made between duplex and contrast angiographic studies.[6] Although we agree that the practice of using duplex as a sole preoperative diagnostic test in patients with focal symptoms of cerebral ischemia may be acceptable, it demands that good quality images be obtained by skilled technicians in certified diagnostic facilities. Few would argue that MRA can provide an array of important information that may help in more precisely defining the best method of treatment in patients with cerebrovascular disease. Unlike duplex imaging, the combination of MRI and MRA can be used to image the brain and screen for pathologic conditions such as cortical ischemia, hemorrhage, tumor, and aneurysms. An additional advantage is that MRA can be used to determine intracranial directional blood flow patterns and to quantitate regional hemispheric blood flow characteristics. A key concept in the application of MR flow information is that the cerebrovasomotor reserve can become quickly exhausted as the resistance arteries of the brain are maximally dilated. This condition is important to recognize because minimal reduction in perfusion pressure may result in cerebral ischemia. Recent clinical experience with the use of acetozolamide (Diamox), a potent intracerebral vasodilator, suggests that its use in combination with 3D TOF assessment of intracranial flow can detect patients who have physiologically important carotid disease, from those that do not. Normally, cerebral flow will increase by at least 30% after a Diamox challenge. A failure to enhance cerebral flow or an observed reduction in hemispheric perfusion after Diamox challenge, suggests that the affected vascular bed is maximally dilated and susceptible to ischemic change should blood pressure or cardiac output drop. In the future, such studies may become important in identifying patients with asymptomatic carotid disease who might most appropriately benefit from carotid endarterectomy procedures.[7]

The most appropriate pretreatment evaluation of patients with symptomatic or high-risk carotid occlusive disease may vary somewhat based on available diagnostic resources. In centers where ultrasonography and high-quality MRA are available, it is possible to avoid use of contrast arteriography in up to 85% of all symptomatic patients. Ultrasonography should be the first test performed in patients with cervical bruits or symptoms suggestive of cerebral ischemia. Doppler ultrasound can be used to establish the presence or absence of significant cervical carotid disease, to differentiate moderate from severe carotid stenosis, and to detect the presence of complete arterial occlusion. In symptomatic patients, the use of 2D TOF MRA in combination with duplex ultrasonography will accurately identify the location and severity of carotid disease in approximately 80% of all symptomatic patients. In those individuals where flow void artifacts cannot be successfully interrogated with 3D TOF imaging, gadolinium contrast enhancement should be performed. A combination of 2D and 3D TOF evaluation with PC imaging of the intracranial circulation is most effective for distinguishing high-grade stenosis from complete internal carotid artery occlusion. We generally reserve the use of contrast arteriography for circumstances where concordance between Doppler ultrasound and MRA cannot be established, where intracranial vascular pathology is suspected, or when duplex suggests the absence of hemodynamically significant cervical carotid disease. Contrast arteriography has better spatial resolution and allows for more precise assessment of minor vessel wall pathology and small vessel disease than is possible by MRA and duplex. In asymptomatic patients with cervical bruits and duplex evidence of borderline or high-grade occlusive disease, we think that 3D TOF with gadolinium will provide the most accurate arteriogram and allow the most probable opportunity for accurate grading of stenosis severity. Doppler alone cannot clearly distinguish borderline intermediate stenoses from high-grade lesions, and it frequently tends to overestimate the severity of stenosis in the presence of coexistent contralateral high-grade stenosis or occlusion.[8]

Although the routine use of preoperative carotid MRA has not been universally accepted, those involved in its research and development are convinced that it will become one of the most important diagnostic imaging tests for evaluation of carotid disease. Standardized protocols for MRA carotid imaging need to be established, and it is essential to conduct institutional quality controls to determine comparative accuracy with X-ray arteriograms and other noninvasive tests. It is likely that MRA will replace routine diagnostic conventional X-ray arteriography to a large extent. In the near future, it is unlikely, however, that MRA will be able to compete with traditional arteriographic methods when it comes to endovascular stent placement, angioplasty, thrombolytic therapy, or intraoperative imaging.

PERIPHERAL VASCULATURE

Magnetic resonance angiography has also assumed a more important role in the diagnosis and management of lower extremity occlusive disease because of its safety, its cost savings, and its ability to precisely image the femoral, popliteal, and distal tibial circulation. Clinical experience strongly suggests that MRA is as sensitive as contrast arteriography for detection of distal occlusive disease and perhaps more sensitive for detection of patent tibial vessels in patients with complex proximal multi-segment occlusive disease.[9] Our initial clinical experience with lower extremity MRA involved patients with non-invasive tests or recurrent clinical symptoms, suggesting impending hemodynamic failure of infrainguinal bypass grafts. This group turned out to be an excellent model for clinical study, because noninvasive testing and contrast arteriography were routinely available for comparison with MRA. Although an absolute correlation of only 75% was initially achieved using MRA, it became quite clear that most of the discrepancies were the result of technical error or poor patient selection. In retrospect, had these problems been understood in our early experience with this technique, primary accuracy rates would have approximated 90%.[10] More recent experience confirms such a high correlation between MRA and contrast arteriography of the lower extremity vessels. Magnetic resonance angiography is well suited for evaluation of extremity blood flow because the host vessels and/or bypass grafts are in superficial tissue planes and are oriented perpendicular to the axial plane of the limbs, thus minimizing in-plane flow signal loss and maximizing flow-related enhancement of flowing blood. Clinical studies confirm that detection of patent distal target vessels can be increased by 7% to 13% if MRA is used.[9] Magnetic resonance angiography is particularly advantageous for evaluating diabetic patients with complex distal vessel occlusive disease and for evaluation of patients with chronic renal failure. We have found that MRA is extremely accurate for localization of disease, for detection of hemodynamically significant lesions, and for distinguishing focal from long-segment stenoses or occlusions. When noninvasive screening tests suggest that distal occlusive disease may be the cause for ischemic limb symptoms, MRA can be used to confirm the diagnosis and to determine an appropriate plan of management. For example, patients with severe claudication or limb-threatening ischemia, and MRA evidence of multisegment stenotic or long-segment arterial occlusion, require bypass surgery. Intra-operative arteriography can confirm patency of host vessels targeted for distal anastomosis. Amputation invariably occurs if gangrene of the foot is associated with a failure of MRA to identify a patent pedal arcade in continuity with open distal tibial vessels. In patients that have short-segment stenoses or occlusions, balloon angioplasty and/or stenting may often be selected as a means of primary treatment. We have found that MRA is very effective in detecting candidates for balloon angioplasty. When MRA is used as a preoperative diagnostic screening test, conventional arteriography can frequently be avoided or used as a therapeutic intervention. In our experience, MRA has been 95% accurate in predicting successful angioplasty candidate selection for treatment of infrainguinal occlusive disease. Selective antegrade arteriography is used for percutaneous transluminal angioplasty of the superficial femoral artery or distal vessel occlusive disease. This approach facilitates access for superficial femoral artery and tibial occlusive lesions and limits the volume of contrast needed.[11]

We have also had great success with use of MRA in the postoperative assessment of patients with distal bypass surgery or angioplasty. When noninvasive tests suggest impending graft failure, MRA has proven very effective in confirming graft patency or occlusion and in identifying the location and severity of occlusive lesions threatening graft function. Interventional management is frequently dictated by the location of the obstructive lesion. Anastomotic strictures or midgraft narrowings of in situ bypass grafts are most commonly associated with scarring or fibrointimal hyperplasia, and require surgical intervention. Host vessel lesions, proximal or distal to the bypass graft, are frequently amenable to balloon angioplasty. In our experience, MRA has proven to be a safe, cost-efficient, outpatient imaging technique that can be used in combination with physical examination and segmental limb pressures to distinguish candidates for balloon angioplasty from those requiring infrainguinal arterial bypass procedures.[11]

Although MRA has assumed growing importance in the clinical assessment of patients with cerebrovascular and lower extremity ischemic symptoms, its role in the evaluation of the thoracoabdominal arterial system has lagged behind because of environmental and technical factors which degrade image quality. These include respiratory and bowel motion, lower signal-to-noise ratios available from body coils compared with head coils, the presence of fatty tissue that creates image artifacts in the maximum intensity projections, and aortic pulsatility that causes ghost artifacts. Early efforts to image aortic branch vessels using 2D TOF and PC techniques demonstrated success in visualization of visceral and renal arteries with ostial or proximal occlusive disease (sensitivity 88%, specificity 96%) but frequently were plagued by overgrading of stenotic lesions because of signal loss in areas of complex flow, and inadequate resolution associated with limited field of view and acquisition matrix size. This made it difficult to identify small accessory renal arteries and to quantify the severity of disease in the distal visceral or hilar branch vessels. Newer imaging protocols, including the use of 3D PC and 2D TOF with PC imaging and breathhold, have improved the sensitivity and specificity for proximal and distal imaging of the aortic branch vessels (sensitivity 89%, specificity 95% for >50% stenoses). However, the most important improvement in thoracoabdominal MRA imaging has resulted from the use of 3D TOF with intravenous gadolinium contrast enhancement.[12, 13] This technique makes it possible to obtain 3D anatomical displays of the thoracic and abdominal aorta using surface-shaded image processing, which is commonly associated with helical spiral CT scans. Three-dimensional contrast MRA covers more territory at high resolution compared with CT-spiral angiography, because of the possibility of a coronal orientation to the MR volume. It avoids exposure to ionizing radiation, does not require use of nephrotoxic contrast agents, can distinguish thrombus from slow flow, and can be used for accurate determination of vessel diameters. These characteristics make it well suited for use in patients with aortic aneurysm disease and, in the future, may be of value in planning endovascular placement of stented grafts.[14–16] The combined use of 3D TOF and paramagnetic contrast agent enhancement has proven quite useful in the evaluation of patients with aortoiliac and distal occlusive disease as well, because it circumvents many of the problems of conventional TOF MRA that result from blood inflow and blood motion characteristics. Three-dimensional TOF

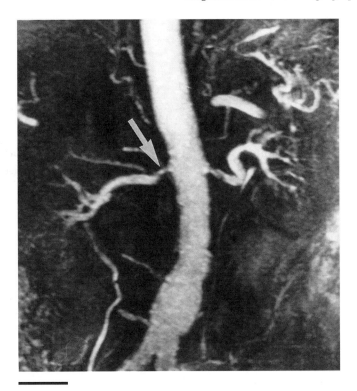

FIGURE 3

Bilateral renal artery stenosis. Full-volume maximum intensity projection (MIP) display of the entire 3-dimensional contrast-enhanced data set. The images demonstrate a severe right renal artery stenosis *(arrow)*, and a moderate proximal left renal artery stenosis. The right stenosis is associated with poststenotic dilatation. Note the extensive aortic atherosclerotic plaque, as well as the aneurysmal dilatation of the infrarenal abdominal aorta. The images were obtained during a 30-second breath-hold after an infusion of 40 mL of gadodiamide.

with gadolinium enhancement reduces the incidence of flow void artifacts, eliminates the problem of in-plane flow, improves spatial resolution, makes it easier to accurately determine the length of stenoses or occlusions, and significantly reduces imaging time requirements. Shortened imaging times allow for patients to breath-hold during MR scans, further enhancing image quality (Fig 3).

The sensitivity and specificity for aortic branch vessel imaging has consequently improved (96% and 98%, respectively). We have used this technique to screen hypertensive patients for renal artery stenosis, to evaluate patients with symptomatic peripheral vascular disease and coexistent renal failure, to evaluate patients with aortic dissections, to assess patients with thoracic and abdominal aortic aneurysms who have hypertension and renal failure, and as a means of postoperative assessment for renal bypass and renal transplant patients.[3]

More recently, we have used PC techniques in combination with gadolinium injection to determine renal artery and corticomedullary blood flow. Because 2D MRI makes it possible to determine vessel cross-section area and because clearance rates for gadolinium can be calculated, volumetric blood flow in the renal artery or in the kidney itself can be determined.[17, 18] Because gadolinium chelates are cleared only by glomerular filtration, it is possible to determine glomerular filtration rates (GFR) by using the following formula:

$$GFR = FF \times RBF \times (1 \times Hct)$$

where FF is filtration fraction, RBF is renal blood flow, and Hct is serum hematocrit.

The glomerular filtration of the gadolinium causes a decrease in the renal vein concentration of this contrast agent, thus increasing the T1 value of venous blood relative to arterial blood. The change in blood relaxation time is used to determine filtration fraction and subsequently glomerular filtration rates. This technique can be performed quickly and allows for independent assessment of each kidney. We have been able to calculate renal blood flow indices which are based on renal artery blood flow volumes and renal organ tissue mass volumes, and have established criteria for normal and abnormal renal perfusion using the following formula:

$$Renal flow volume index = RBF \div Renal volume$$
$$(normal, \geq 2 \text{ mL/min/cc renal mass}).$$

This information may be of particular value in the postoperative assessment of patients with renal artery reconstructions and renal transplantation. This test may ultimately enable physicians to distinguish prerenal ischemic events from cortical dysfunction in postoperative kidney transplant recipients who have elevated blood pressure and progressive azotemia. Our current experience suggests that gadolinium-enhanced MRA can provide a safe and accurate alternative to ionic contrast–based arteriography or CT imaging of the aortic branch vessels. It can be used to identify patients that may benefit from balloon angioplasty or surgical reconstruction of renal arteries, it can provide important information regarding the relationship between the neck of an abdominal aortic aneurysm and the renal or visceral arteries, it can be used to diagnose and categorize aortic dissections, and may serve as an important alternative to contrast arteriography in evaluation of peripheral vascular disease in patients with impaired renal function. The next major advance in MR technology will probably be in real-time imaging, which may allow for its potential use in endovascular procedures.

REFERENCES

1. Anderson CM, Edelman RR, Turski PA: *Clinical Magnetic Resonance Angiography.* New York, Raven Press, 1993.
2. Turnipseed WD, Kennell TW, Turski PA, et al: Combined use of duplex imaging and magnetic resonance angiography for evaluation of patients with symptomatic ipsilateral high-grade carotid stenosis. *J Vasc Surg* 17:832–840, 1993.
3. Prince MR, Grist TM, Debatin JF: *3D Contrast MR Angiography.* Berlin, Springer-Verlag, 1997.
4. Turnipseed WD, Kennell TW, Turski PA, et al: Magnetic resonance angiography and duplex imaging: Noninvasive tests for selecting symptomatic carotid endarterectomy candidates. *Surgery* 114:643–649, 1993.
5. Polak JF, Kalina P, Donaldson MC, et al: Carotid endarterectomy: Preoperative evaluation of candidates with combined Doppler sonography and MR angiography. *Radiology* 186:333–338, 1993.
6. Moore WS, Mohr JP, Najafi H, et al: Carotid endarterectomy: Practice guidelines. *J Vasc Surg* 15:469–479, 1992.
7. Turski PA, Levine R, Turnipseed W, et al: MR angiography flow analysis: Neurovascular applications. *Magn Reson Imaging Clin North Am* 3:541–555, 1995.
8. Strandness DE Jr: Carotid endarterectomy without angiography, in Yao JST, Pearce WH (eds): *Progress in Vascular Surgery.* Stamford, Conn: Appleton & Lange, 1997, pp 99–108.
9. Baum RA, Rutter CM, Sunshine JH, et al: Multi-center trial to evaluate vascular magnetic resonance angiography of the lower extremity. *JAMA* 274:875–880, 1995.
10. Turnipseed WD, Sproat IA: A preliminary experience with use of magnetic resonance angiography in assessment of failing lower extremity bypass grafts. *Surgery* 112:664–669, 1992.
11. Hoch JR, Tullis MJ, Kennell TW, et al: Use of magnetic resonance angiography for the preoperative evaluation of patients with infrainguinal arterial occlusive disease. *J Vasc Surg* 23:792–801, 1996.
12. Prince MR, Yucel EK, Kaufman JA, et al: Dynamic gadolinium-enhanced three-dimensional abdominal MR arteriography. *J Magn Reson Imaging* 3:877–881, 1993.

13. Prince MR: Gadolinium-enhanced MR aortography. *Radiology* 191: 155–164, 1994.

14. Petersen MJ, Cambria RP, Kaufman JA, et al: Magnetic resonance angiography in the preoperative evaluation of abdominal aortic aneurysms. *J Vasc Surg* 21:891–899, 1995.

15. Prince MR, Narasimham DL, Stanley JC, et al: Gadolinium-enhanced magnetic resonance angiography of abdominal aortic aneurysms. *J Vasc Surg* 21:656–669, 1995.

16. Durham JR, Hackworth CA, Tober JC, et al: Magnetic resonance angiography in the preoperative evaluation of abdominal aortic aneurysms. *Am J Surg* 166:173–178, 1993.

17. Niendorf ER, Grist TM, Frayne R: Rapid measurement of Gd-DTPA extraction fraction in a dialysis system using echo-planar imaging. *Med Phys* 24:1907–1913, 1997.

18. Niendorf ER, Grist TM, Lee Jr FT, et al. Rapid in vivo measurement of single kidney extraction fraction and glomerular filtration rate with MRI imaging. *Radiology,* 206:791–798, 1998.

CHAPTER 12

Endoscopic Techniques for Harvesting the Greater Saphenous Vein

Jae-Sung Cho, M.D.
Fellow, Division of Vascular Surgery, Mayo Clinic, Rochester, Minnesota

Peter Gloviczki, M.D.
Professor of Surgery, Mayo Medical School, Vice Chair, Division of
Vascular Surgery, Mayo Clinic, Rochester, Minnesota

A utologous saphenous vein is the most frequently used conduit for coronary and infrainguinal arterial reconstructions. Dissection of the greater saphenous vein (GSV) is traditionally performed through one long or several shorter skin incisions. However, vein harvesting can be complicated by a wide spectrum of wound problems (Table 1). Although major complications are infrequent, delayed wound healing or wound infections frequently requiring prolonged hospital care have been reported to occur in up to 44% of patients who have undergone GSV harvesting using traditional surgical techniques.[1–3] One prospective trial revealed preoperative predictors of poor wound healing to be female sex, diabetes mellitus, peripheral arterial occlusive disease, obesity, hematocrit less than 35%, and left ventricular end-diastolic pressure greater than 15 mm Hg.[1]

Morbidity associated with leg incisions was recognized as early as 1906 by Charles H. Mayo, who developed an external vein stripper to remove varicose veins without long skin incisions.[1–4] It is remarkable that current minimally invasive surgical techniques use a modified Mayo stripper (pigtail dissector) as the main dissecting instrument to mobilize the saphenous vein for harvest under endoscopic control (Fig 1). Experience using different endoscopic instrumentations to harvest the GSV has rapidly increased in recent years (Fig 2).[5–9] In this chapter, we describe the technique of endoscopic saphenous vein harvesting using the Ethicon-Endosurgery

TABLE 1.
Complications of
Greater Saphenous
Vein Harvest

Wound infection
Cellulitis
Lymphangitis
Skin necrosis
Wound dehiscence
Lymphorrhea
Lymphocele
Seroma
Hematoma
Abscess
Saphenous neuralgia
Paresthesia
Graft failure
Limb amputation

Inc. instrumentation, the method with which we are most familiar. We will also discuss current indications, advantages, and early complications of the endoscopic techniques.

TECHNIQUE OF ENDOSCOPIC VEIN HARVESTING

The principal instrument is a disposable subcutaneous retractor that incorporates a 5-mm straight or a 30-degree angled endoscopic camera for viewing. This retractor is available in two different sizes. The endoscopic instruments include a pigtail dissector (a modified Mayo vein stripper; Fig 1), an endoscopic clip applier (5-mm Allport Clip applier), and endoscopic scissors (Ethicon Endo-Surgery Inc., Cincinnati, Ohio). Two video monitors are set up at opposite sides of the operating table for comfortable viewing by both the surgeon and the first assistant. The monitors are placed as close to the table as possible, and the operating room lights are dimmed during dissection for easy viewing.

The patient is placed supine with the legs prepared circumferentially with the leg in a "frog-leg" position. An incision along the groin crease is made beginning at the medial border of the common femoral artery and extending medially 2.5 cm. A longer, longitudinal incision is made only if the femoral artery also has to be

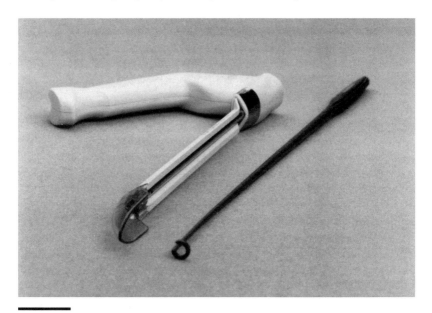

FIGURE 1.
Left, endoscopic dissector/retractor with a port for a 5- × 300-mm video-scopic lens. **Right,** a pigtail dissector (a modified Mayo vein stripper).

exposed as the site of proximal anastomosis of a femorodistal graft. The saphenofemoral junction is identified, and all tributaries to the GSV are ligated proximally and distally. It is better not to divide these tributaries yet, because they are helpful in stabilizing the GSV and enabling easier advancement of the endoscopic retractor in a distal direction. A subcutaneous tunnel is developed caudally over the anterior surface of the GSV, while exposure is provided by a hand-held narrow Richardson retractor. This is replaced by the endoscopic retractor containing the 5-mm videoscope (Fig 1), which is then advanced distally to dissect and retract the tissues along the anterior surface of the vein. A gentle upward pressure has to be applied on the retractor during this part of the procedure not only to advance it easier in a distal direction, but also to avoid injury to the saphenous vein by stripping its adventitia. Tributaries of the saphenous vein are located usually in the medial and lateral aspects, and only a few anterior branches are present on the thigh. All tributaries are clipped and divided as soon as they are visualized by the endoscope to avoid avulsion of these as the retractor is advanced distally. Because bleeding through transected tributaries of the GSV is usually insignificant because of spasm of the vein,

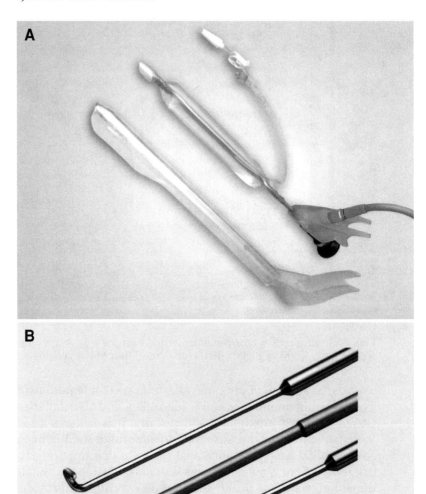

FIGURE 2.
A, endoscopic instrumentation with balloon dissector, video camera, and a rigid plastic retractor from General Surgical Innovations. **B,** reusable dissecting instruments for endoscopic vein harvest.

only very large tributaries need to be double clipped before division. Only one lateral clip is placed on most tributaries, which are then divided several millimeters away from the GSV to allow safe ligation after removal of the vein from the tunnel (Fig 3). Of critical importance, the GSV must not be held under great tension during dissection to avoid adventitial and endothelial damage.

Once the limits of the retractor are reached (30 cm), the pigtail dissector is inserted to free up the vein circumferentially (Fig 4). Additional lateral and any posterior tributaries are dissected, clipped, and divided (Fig 3). Because clips were placed only laterally on the tributaries, the pigtail dissector can be advanced over the GSV without danger of vein injury. Nevertheless, smaller tributaries are frequently avulsed during dissection, rendering in situ bypass rather difficult to perform because of bleeding in the tunnel through these sites.

When the entire length of the exposed vein is mobilized, which usually is not the full length of the thigh, additional distal incisions are made to insert the scope for further dissections. If the popliteal artery is the site of the distal anastomosis, a standard longitudinal incision should be made over the saphenous vein at that area. The vein has been mapped and marked preoperatively with duplex scanning. Even if the popliteal artery was not to be exposed, a longer incision at the knee level, where multiple genicular tributaries join the GSV, is justified to minimize vein injury. The dissection can be continued distally on the calf using the technique described, although small venous tributaries in the calf are frequently encountered, and a more time-consuming dissection is necessary to avoid vein injury. The adjacent saphenous nerve should be protected at the knee and the calf during vein dissection.

Upon completion of the vein dissection, the proximal end of the saphenous vein is divided first, after placing a vascular clamp on the vein at the saphenofemoral confluence. The proximal cut end of the GSV is oversewn with 4-0 polypropylene running suture. The distal end can be occluded either by clips or ligated by an Endo-loop (Ethicon Endo-Surgery Inc., Cincinnati, Ohio). A small incision can also be made in the calf to ligate the vein at its distal end.

After removal, the vein is cannulated through the distal end and distended with heparinized saline/papaverine solution (our vein solution contains 1,000 units of heparin sodium and 30 mg of papaverine in 400 mL of normal saline). Inflation over arterial pressure (120 mm Hg) is avoided by using a syringe with a pressure

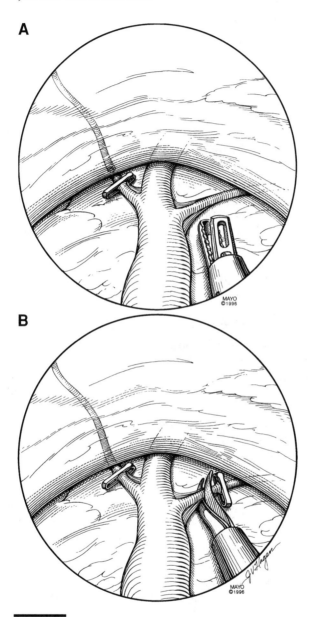

FIGURE 3.

After the side branches are clipped with endoscopic clip applier on the side of the body **(A)**, they are divided with endoscopic scissors on the side of the vein **(B)**. Venospasm and competent valves minimize blood loss.

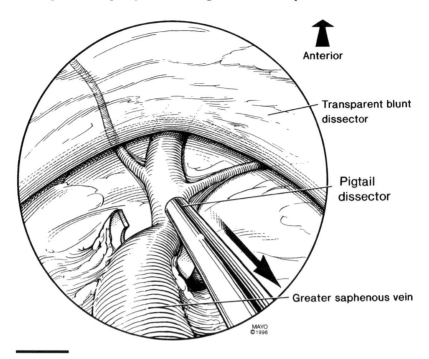

FIGURE 4.

The anterior surface of the saphenous vein has been dissected using endoscopic dissector. The vein is encircled with the open circle of the pigtail dissector and gently dissected from surrounding soft tissue, and the branches identified.

gauge. Previously transected tributaries are ligated with 3-0 or 4-0 silk ties, and any tears are repaired with 7-0 monofilament polypropylene sutures.

The tunnel is inspected at the end of the procedure for evidence of active bleeding or hematomas. Small bleeders are cauterized and larger vessels occluded by endoclips. The wounds are closed in layers and if arterial reconstruction was not done on the same extremity, the leg is wrapped with an ACE bandage to decrease chances of postoperative bleeding.

DISCUSSION

Wound complications after harvesting of the GSV for arterial conduit can present significant problems and may result in prolonged hospitalization for both cardiac and peripheral vascular surgery patients. Various techniques including "skip" incisions with intervening skin "bridges" have been proposed to minimize wound problems. The "skip" incision technique has shown a reduction in wound complication rate in one study from 21.7% to 8.8%.[10] In a prospective review of GSV harvest using a modified Mayo vein stripper and multiple small incisions for 2,439 coronary artery bypasses, no major wound complications were reported, and minor wound problems occurred in only 0.9% of patients.[11] Such data justify attempts to avoid skin incisions in the leg using minimally invasive, endoscopic techniques for saphenous vein harvest.

Early reports of endoscopic procurement of the GSV described a reduced rate of wound complications. Lumsden et al. observed only three wound complications after endoscopic removal of the GSV in 30 limbs. Two of these patients had cautery burns, and one patient had injury to the saphenous vein.[6] In a prospective series of 68 consecutive GSVs harvested for lower extremity revascularization, Jordan et al. reported a wound complication rate of 8.8%.[5] This was significantly lower than the 24.3% wound complication rate observed using standard open harvesting techniques.[1] No graft failure or graft harvest–related wound complications were noted.[5] Dimitri et al., using subcutaneous extraluminal vein dissector with multiple small incisions in 428 patients, observed no major wound complications requiring prolonged hospitalization.[8] In another study, endovascular in situ saphenous vein bypass reduced the wound complication rate to 3.7%.[12] All studies using endoscopic harvesting techniques emphasize improvement in patient comfort, early mobility, decreased length of hospital stay, and superior cosmetic results. Decreased wound complications are associated with a shortened length of hospital stay as reported by Jordan and associates, who noted that only 6 of 65 patients required prolonged hospitalization because of wound problems.[5] Saphenous neuralgia has been reported to occur in as many as 22% of patients who underwent femoropopliteal bypass in one series.[13] While endovascular harvesting does not seem to eliminate nerve injury, it appears to reduce the risk of saphenous neuralgia.[5]

Another issue that must be considered in evaluating endoscopic harvesting is the risk of vein injury, which may reduce long-term graft patency. Vein injuries requiring vein patch angioplasty occurred in two patients in Jordan and associates' series, and one of the veins thrombosed 5 months after operation.[5] The primary patency rate of femoropopliteal bypasses was 63.5% and the secondary patency rate was 83.5% after a mean follow-up of 7.9 months (range 1–24 months).

Several studies have investigated the effects of minimally invasive GSV harvest on morphology and function of the veins. Meldrum-Hanna et al. demonstrated preservation of intima by scanning electron microscopy (SEM) and observed a 93% graft patency rate at 10 days after surgery.[11] In another histologic study of vein samples using both light microscopy and SEM, preservation of endothelial architecture, normal cell cohesion, and normal intercellular junctional gaps were observed.[8] Functional studies from the Mayo Clinic of porcine venous endothelium after endoscopic harvest showed comparable non–receptor-mediated relaxations to those harvested with the standard method,[14] and SEM did not show significant differences in endothelial integrity between the two.

Endoscopic saphenous vein harvest requires more operative time than traditional open procedures. Lumsden and associates reported the average time for harvest to be 1.25 hours.[6] However, the initial learning curve is steep, and in our experience, dissection time can be reduced to 30–45 minutes for groin to knee length. Jordan and colleagues reported a dissection time of 0.9 cm per minute using the same technique. When skin closure time after standard technique is considered, this time frame is acceptable, particularly for those at high risk for wound complications.

CONCLUSION

Endoscopic harvest of saphenous vein is an effective technique that can be easily learned. Correctly done, it is atraumatic to the vein, with preservation of venous endothelial functions and structural integrity. This technique is not limited by anatomical location of reconstruction, and thus can be used for coronary artery bypass grafting, lower extremity bypass, or for renal artery reconstructions. Patients' discomfort and wound complications are also reduced, and cosmetic results are improved. Endoscopic harvesting of the GSV should definitely be considered for patients undergoing coronary artery bypass grafting who have peripheral arterial ischemia, and for those undergoing peripheral vascular reconstruction who are at high risk for wound complications.

REFERENCES

1. Utley JR, Thomason ME, Wallace DJ, et al: Preoperative correlates of impaired wound healing after saphenous vein excision. *J Thorac Cardiovasc Surg* 98:147–149, 1989.

2. DeLaria GA, Hunter JA, Goldin MD, et al: Leg wound complications associated with coronary revascularization. *J Thorac Cardiovasc Surg* 81:403–407, 1981.

3. Reifsnyder T, Bandyk D, Seabrook G, et al: Wound complications of the in situ saphenous vein bypass technique. *J Vasc Surg* 15:843–850, 1992.

4. Mayo CH: Treatment of varicose veins. *Surg Gynecol Obstet* 2:385–388, 1906.

5. Jordan WD, Voellinger DC, Schroeder PT, et al: Video-assisted saphenous vein harvest: The evolution of a new technique. *J Vasc Surg* 26:405–414, 1997.

6. Lumsden AB, Eaves FF, Ofenloch JC, et al: Subcutaneous, video-assisted saphenous vein harvest: Report of the first 30 cases. *Cardiovasc Surg* 4:771–776, 1996.

7. Cable DG, Dearani JA: Endoscopic saphenous vein harvesting: Minimally invasive video-assisted saphenectomy. *Ann Thorac Surg* 64:1183–1185, 1997.

8. Dimitri WR, West IE, Williams BT: A quick and atraumatic method of autologous vein harvesting using the subcutaneous extraluminal dissector. *J Cardiovasc Surg* 28:103–111, 1987.

9. Earle DB, Karanfilian RG, Yang HK, et al: Minimally invasive saphenous vein harvest in peripheral vascular bypass procedures. *Surg Rounds* 21:66–77, 1998.

10. Wengrovitz M, Atnip RG, Gifford RRM, et al: Wound complications of autogenous subcutaneous infrainguinal arterial bypass surgery: Predisposing factors and management. *J Vasc Surg* 11:156–163, 1990.

11. Meldrum-Hanna W, Ross D, Johnson D, et al: An improved technique for long saphenous vein harvesting for coronary revascularizaiton. *Ann Thorac Surg* 42:90–92 1986.

12. Rosenthal D, Dickson C, Rodriguez FJ, et al: Infrainguinal endovascular in situ saphenous vein bypass: Ongoing results. *J Vasc Surg* 20:389–395, 1994.

13. Adar R, Meyer E, Zweig A: Saphenous neuralgia: A complication of vascular reconstructions below the knee. *Ann Surg* 190:609–613, 1979.

14. Cable DG, Dearani JA, Pfeifer EA, et al: Minimally invasive saphenous vein harvesting: Functional and histologic analysis of endothelial integrity and early clinical experience. *Ann Thorac Surg,* in press.

CHAPTER 13

Management of the Thrombosed Infrainguinal Vein Graft

Daniel B. Walsh, M.D.
Professor of Surgery, Section of Vascular Surgery, Dartmouth-Hitchcock Medical Center, Lebanon, New Hampshire

M anagement of the patient whose infrainguinal vein graft has thrombosed is a complex therapeutic challenge. Patient survival and limb salvage depend on rapid decisions regarding etiology, technique, and timing of multiple possible therapies, as well as assessment of complex patient risk factors. To further complicate this difficult circumstance, few vascular surgeons have frequent current experience with the many situations possible in patients whose infrainguinal grafts have failed. During the last 30 years, the results of infrainguinal revascularization have consistently improved. Despite this, however, 20% to 30% of patients will have graft failure within 5 years of their initial operation. Technical advances have not only improved results but also have increased the pool of patients in whom limb salvage is thought possible.[1, 2] This discussion attempts to briefly summarize, from the accumulated experience of the discipline of vascular surgery, a reliable set of therapeutic guidelines for the most common among the many possible circumstances where patients are seen with thrombosis of their infrainguinal vein grafts.

GENERAL CONSIDERATIONS

Regardless of the specific circumstances of the failed graft, several factors, possibly contributing to any graft failure, should be investigated. If not previously known, the patient's coagulation status should be determined. Graft thrombosis at any time after placement can be the consequence of a previously unrecognized hypercoagulable state.[3] Blood should be sent immediately (before anticoagulation) for measurement of standard coagulation parameters, as well as functional activated protein C resistance, antithrombin III, and protein S. Other less likely causes of hypercoagulability leading to graft thrombosis, such as sepsis or increased blood viscosity from dehydration or polycythemia, can easily be ruled out with physical examination and routine hematologic screening. Acute or chronic cardiac decompensation is another uncommon cause of graft thrombosis that can be rapidly diagnosed during the admission examination and confirmed with ECG or echocardiography as indicated. This cardiac assessment will also be critical in assessing the risks associated with the various possible therapeutic options.

Consideration should be given to systemically anticoagulating the patient at presentation or at the first practical opportunity. As mentioned above, coagulation studies should be drawn before initiation of anticoagulation therapy. Determination of the need for and the timing of operation should also be made, because anticoagulation should be delayed long enough to institute epidural anesthesia if this is clinically desirable. If immediate operation is not required or epidural anesthesia is contraindicated, systemic heparin anticoagulation should be instituted to inhibit propagation of the thrombus.

Neurologic status at the time of presentation is a primary determinant of the timing of therapy. If there is no neurologic compromise, diagnostic or therapeutic maneuvers, which may take considerable time, can be attempted. As the level of neurologic function deteriorates from dysesthesia to paralysis, the requirement for rapid resolution of the situation increases, and the time available for lengthy diagnostic or therapeutic measures outside of the operating room, correspondingly decreases.

ETIOLOGY

The first step toward successful therapy of a failed infrainguinal vein graft is accurate determination of the cause for the thrombosis. Figure 1 lists the five elements whose optimization is required for effective graft function. For any graft to function, blood flow into the graft (inflow) must be at systemic pressure with the graft patent. Any gradient between the site of the proximal graft anastomosis and central systemic pressure demonstrates the existence of a significant proximal arterial stenosis. Few grafts will remain patent and no revascularizations will long succeed if their inflow is significantly compromised.

Inflow

Outflow

Conduit

Technique

Coagulation State

FIGURE 1.
Critical elements for graft function.

Without adequate outflow, the best of grafts will likely fail because flow will be too low to prevent thrombus formation. The quality of the graft's outflow is an extremely difficult characteristic to define or measure. Many runoff beds composed of only a few small vessels seem too sparse to support a graft over a long period. Yet, no arteriographic criteria have been found to be reliable predictors of long-term graft patency. As an example, Figure 2 shows a runoff bed based on the anterior lateral malleolar artery. The dorsalis pedis and posterior tibial arteries are not seen. This graft has been patent for more than 18 months. Measurement of outflow bed resistance has been shown to be predictive of graft failure.[4] However, most surgeons find these methods cumbersome and lacking in the level of accuracy needed for the confident recommendation for conversion of a revascularization attempt to a primary amputation.

A pressure gradient measured over the course of the graft is evidence of significant abnormalities within the conduit whose presence may cause early graft thrombosis.[5] These abnormalities must be identified (see below) and rectified if an enduring revascularization is to be achieved.

The time from initial revascularization to patient presentation with recurrent limb ischemia is the single most important characteristic that aids in the determination of the etiology of graft failure. Most surgeons separate graft failures into three temporal categories: early (within 30 days of placement), intermediate (30 days to 2 years), and late (greater than 2 years).

EARLY GRAFT FAILURE

Despite maturation of infrainguinal vein graft revascularization techniques, 5% to 10% of grafts will fail within 30 days of place-

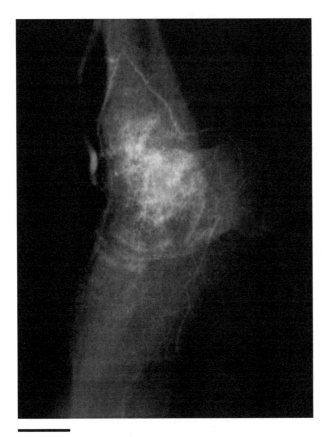

FIGURE 2.
An example of a runoff bed based on the anterior lateral malleolar artery.
The dorsalis pedis and posterior tibial arteries are not seen.

ment.[6] Determination of the response to early graft failure begins
during the latter stages of the initial revascularization. Technical
adequacy of the bypass must be confirmed before closure. This is
accomplished most commonly with intraoperative arteriography
and pencil Doppler examination or, increasingly, with color-flow
duplex ultrasonography. The advantages of these techniques are
their simplicity and wide availability. A patent graft with no evidence of significant arteriovenous fistulas, retained valve cusps, or
anastomotic problems is likely to function well for a long time.
When the graft is demonstrated to fill the desired runoff and gen-
erate an audible pulse that is significantly augmented by graft patency, the surgeon feels assured of long-term graft function. However, intraoperative duplex scanning at the conclusion of an

infrainguinal revascularization has identified abnormalities ranging in frequency of occurrence from 14% to 48%, depending upon the revascularization technique used.[7] Confirmation of systemic pressure at the proximal anastomosis with no loss of pressure at the distal anastomosis once graft patency has been established is also reassuring. Use of angioscopy in vein preparation and evaluation of the vein conduit reduces the number of conduit-related technical problems.[8–10] For example, since routine valve lysis using angioscopic guidance was instituted at Dartmouth-Hitchcock Medical Center (DHMC), valvulatome injury as a cause of early vein graft failure has vanished from our series.

Using these techniques to confirm technical adequacy at bypass completion, the likelihood that a technical flaw has caused graft failure is low. In 1990, when we had begun to use several of these techniques, a review of our institutional experience demonstrated that technical errors accounted for only 25% of our early graft failures.[11] During the past 8 years, the number of graft failures in our series caused by errors in technique has continued to decline sharply. Thus, confirmation of technical adequacy now allows a prospective qualitative determination at the completion of each bypass of the likelihood of graft failure due to the quality of conduit or runoff. This evaluation greatly simplifies further therapeutic decision making. If a graft fails that has been constructed using the only available autogenous vein and runoff vessel, and has no evidence of anastomosis or conduit problem, early amputation will speed most patients toward their best available outcome. In such patients, further reoperative attempts at thrombectomy, anastomosis improvement, conduit replacement, or runoff substitution are only likely to increase morbidity, mortality, and expense, with little improvement in limb salvage.[12]

After initial graft thrombosis, however, the first question to answer is, "Can the graft be salvaged?" Because this first attempt at bypass uses the best conduit and target vessel, most surgeons would answer "Yes." Once the determination to proceed has been made, then the decision is whether surgical or chemical thrombectomy must be performed. The choice of which technique to use is difficult because the results of both are discouraging in the early postoperative period

Patency of thrombosed grafts after attempted lysis during the early postoperative period ranges from 15% to 20% after 1 year.[13, 14] Time since initial vein graft placement has been found to be predictive of both short- and long-term graft patencies after lysis. The more recently placed the graft, the less likely there will be any success with lytic therapy. This is particularly true among patients with diabetes. In our own series, no patient with diabetes and a recently placed graft achieved secondary graft patency with thrombolysis. Forty-four percent of patients successfully treated with thrombolysis required early amputation. If thrombolysis failed, the amputation rate rose to 69%.

Current techniques for catheter thrombolysis usually include guide wire passage through the thrombus, followed by the infusion of 250,000 units of urokinase through the clot. This is followed by infusion of 2,000 units per minute of urokinase within and at the proximal tip of the thrombus. After 12–24 hours of intraclot thrombolysis, arteriographic assessment is repeated. During this process the patient is anticoagulated with heparin. Lysis is continued until the clot is completely dissolved. At that point, detailed arteriography of the extremity should be performed to determine the cause of failure and possible therapeutic options. If no evidence of lysis is demonstrated after 4–6 hours, or if lysis has not succeeded within 48 hours, little further benefit is likely to occur and other therapies should be initiated.

The results of surgical thrombectomy, even with an adjunctive procedure such as patch angioplasty of the distal anastomosis, are uniformly poor. Robinson et al. reported a cumulative secondary patency rate of 37% at 1 year.[12] In this series, 26% of patients required amputation within 1 month of graft thrombectomy. The incidence of patients requiring amputation rose to 41% at 1 year. The results of surgical thrombectomy significantly improved if, at exploration, a technical problem such as a twist in the graft or a retained valve cusp was discovered. In our experience, long-term patency of grafts that thrombosed because of correctable technical problems approached that of grafts in which no complications occurred in the early postoperative period. However, the number of technical flaws causing graft failures has decreased dramatically with improved techniques of graft placement.[12]

The technique for surgical thrombectomy is straightforward. Incisions over proximal, distal, and any interval anastomoses should be reopened. Open thrombectomy protects delicate suture lines from catheter tip trauma and permits transgraft, catheter-based assessment of inflow with measurement of intragraft pressures. A pressure differential of greater than 10 mm Hg from upper extremity or more proximal aorta, compared with pressures obtained at the proximal anastomosis or within the graft after thrombectomy, should focus attention to that particular segment of the circulation. Arteriography, angioscopy, and ultrasound can then be used to confirm the adequacy of the thrombectomy and identify causes for the pressure decrease. Once the identified problems have been corrected, demonstration of technical accuracy of the repair as well as graft function (see above) should be repeated to guarantee optimal graft function. In this difficult circumstance, we maintain systemic anticoagulation throughout the immediate postoperative period and after discharge unless otherwise contraindicated. This prolonged anticoagulation is an attempt to overcome the thrombogenicity we believe innate in a vein graft after thrombosis and balloon thrombectomy.[15]

Our own practice has been to immediately reexplore any patient whose graft has failed after initial revascularization if we have a high expectation of good graft function. We have not found thrombolysis useful in this situation because of the time required for lysis and the additional risk of bleeding during thrombolysis. In this group of patients, thrombectomy, anticoagulation, and repair of any possible technical problems appear to achieve the best results.

In at least 50% of the patients explored for early graft failure, no cause for failure will be found.[16] In these desperate circumstances where a correctable problem has not been found and we are unwilling to implicate poor conduit or disadvantaged runoff as a cause for the thrombosis, we have placed a 20-gauge polyethylene catheter in a convenient proximal side branch of the vein graft after thrombectomy. Through this catheter, nitroglycerin (0.05 μg/min) and heparin (10 units/min) are infused with the patient in the postanesthesia recovery unit or the ICU. This is an attempt to counteract presumed but undocumented thrombogenicity within the "revascularization," whether related to runoff spasm or graft harvest trauma. These catheters are usually removed at the bedside or in the operating room after 24–36 hours of infusion. Eight of 10 grafts so treated have remained patent during a mean follow-up of 17 months.

If all measures at diagnosis and treatment of infrainguinal vein graft thrombosis in the early postoperative period fail, only two options remain. The first is expectant therapy combined with anticoagulation. This will likely lead to amputation, although limb loss is not inevitable. If adequate autogenous vein remains, particularly if there are target vessels with runoff of good quality, repeat vein bypass often yields gratifying results.[17] (see below)

INTERMITTENT AND LATE GRAFT FAILURES

Despite the tradition of dividing graft failures into intermediate, commonly attributed to intimal hyperplasia, and late, usually associated with progression of atherosclerosis, we consider both groups together because, in our opinion, this distinction is less useful for planning therapy. In dealing with patients whose grafts have failed later than 1 month, all the above-mentioned general considerations for evaluation and patient therapy still apply. The major differences in treatment strategy focus on the disappearance of technical error from the list of potential causes of graft failure, the improvement of the results of thrombolysis, and the increased difficulty of the surgical dissection of previously operated vessels.

Since time from graft placement predicts results of thrombolysis in thrombosed vein grafts, the longer a graft has been in place, the greater the likelihood the patient and graft patency will benefit from thrombolysis. Factors critical in predicting success appear to be graft age of approximately 1 year or older and the absence of diabetes. In the DHMC series, only 1 of 15 failed grafts (7%) among patients with diabetes had a patent graft 1 year after successful thrombolysis. In patients without diabetes whose grafts had been patent for at least 12 months before thrombosis, 44% of patients were alive with patent grafts 2 years after thrombolysis.

Once patency has been restored, the likelihood that further endovascular or surgical therapy will be required to ensure long-term graft patency exceeds 85%. Therapeutic options include balloon angioplasty of intragraft or juxta-anastomotic stenoses, open vein patch angioplasty, or interposition vein bypass. Although the results of these techniques used to maintain patency of threatened grafts (so-called primary assisted patency) are not comparable to results obtained in failed grafts patent after thrombolysis, experience in this threatened group is much larger and provides a significant body of data from which useful direction can be drawn.

Surgical treatment of hemodynamically significant vein graft lesions achieved patency at 21 months in 86% of grafts, whereas the patency rate of lesions treated with percutaneous angioplasty was 42%.[18] This difference is particularly noteworthy because the surgical group, in the opinion of the authors, had more extensive disease than patients treated percutaneously. Other groups have recently reported significantly better results for angioplasty of graft stenoses.[19] Excellent results for either technique have been published. We believe percutaneous transluminal angioplasty is best used to maintain graft patency until after operative repair can be undertaken, to treat straightforward short stenoses that are difficult to approach surgically, or to dilate critical stenoses in patients with medical contraindications to anesthesia or surgery.

Selection of patch angioplasty vs. interposition graft for repair of graft lesions should be made using lesion location and appearance, availability of usable autogenous vein, and the surgeon's preference as determinants. A detailed review of an experience with both techniques demonstrates that results are similar.[20] Our bias is that removal of the hyperplastic intimal lesion via interposition grafting should lead to better results. However, two additional anastomoses within the graft carry their own complication rate. Factors influencing the decision include lesion length and appearance, as well as the quality and availability of autogenous vein. For juxta-anastomotic problems in the distal graft, exposure of the distal target artery beyond the initial anastomosis is technically simpler and less morbid than reoperating at the initial anastomotic site. This option is only possible if suitable lengths of autogenous vein adequate for bypass graft extension are available.

The optimal autogenous vein conduit for replacement of a short segment of vein graft is a segment of remaining ipsilateral saphenous vein or lesser saphenous vein. Interposition of a segment of contralateral greater saphenous or arm vein to provide a short interposition should be avoided to preserve these longer conduits for other uses.

In the group of patients whose older grafts are demonstrated after successful lysis to have had diffuse deterioration, and in patients who have diabetes or whose grafts have failed in less than 1 year, we would forego thrombolysis because of the small likelihood of achieving any significant secondary graft patency. For these groups, repeat bypass has the greatest chance of achieving successful long-term revascularization. Of course, quality distal target vessels and adequate autogenous vein conduit are mandatory if repeat bypass is to be attempted.

Figure 3 compares long-term graft patencies achieved by all techniques of graft salvage, from repeat bypass and graft revision to thrombolysis under the best of circumstances. Despite the obvious benefit of repeat bypass in this comparison, it is important to remember that these patient groups are only superficially comparable. In this series, conduit availability, condition of runoff, coagulation status, and other important circumstances are either not comparable or not known. For example, in our own patients undergoing thrombolysis, repeat bypass was possible in only 1 of 44 patients. This emphasizes again the complexity of these patients and the importance of understanding the condition of all 5 elements (Fig 1) needed for successful bypass at the time of initial

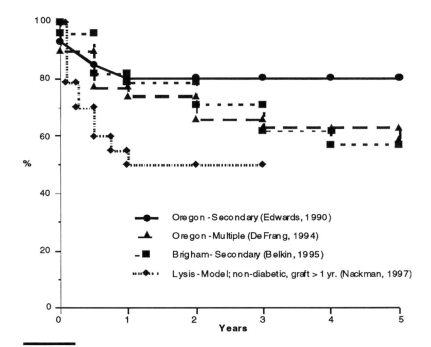

FIGURE 3.

Comparison of long-term patency of secondary bypass, initial bypass salvage vein surgery, and thrombolysis among the patient group with the best results.

bypass completion and at the time of thrombosis when salvage options are being considered.

Conduit availability and selection is another good example of the complexity of the decision making when a vein graft has failed. The contralateral greater saphenous vein has long been thought to be the optimal conduit for bypass when the ipsilateral greater saphenous vein is not available because of disease or prior use. Concern that the donor leg might require bypass in the future or that the saphenous vein might be required for coronary artery bypass has been outweighed by the immediate need and the belief that the reduced survival of these patients makes the need for future bypass elsewhere unlikely. Examination of the infrainguinal bypass experience at DHMC revealed that 20% of our patients required contralateral lower-extremity revascularization at a mean of 31 months after initial ipsilateral bypass.[21] The intervention rate in our patients by life table analysis was relatively linear at 6% per year. Eighty-three percent of these interventions were contralateral infrainguinal vein bypass. Factors that predicted the need for intervention were younger age, presence of diabetes, overt coronary artery disease, and lower contralateral ankle-brachial index at the time of initial ipsilateral revascularization.

In patients with only unilateral lower-extremity atherosclerosis severe enough to require operation, the likelihood of future contralateral intervention is less than 10% during the next 5 years. Thus, contralateral saphenous vein, the optimal bypass conduit, should be used to revascularize the contralateral leg in older patients with atherosclerosis isolated to one limb. In this patient group, the surgeon can proceed, confident that the requirement for the use of this vein elsewhere is very unlikely. Unfortunately, only 8% of patients who typically require infrainguinal revascularization have only isolated unilateral lower-extremity atherosclerosis. Rather, 32% of our infrainguinal bypass patients have both diabetes and coronary artery disease. Thirty-one percent of these patients required intervention for ischemia of their contralateral leg within 5 years of their initial infrainguinal revascularization. Twenty-two percent of our patients have diabetes, coronary artery disease, and low contralateral ankle-brachial index—half of these patients required later contralateral intervention. Therefore, we believe that the selection of bypass conduit when ipsilateral greater saphenous vein is not available is complex.

Arm vein, deemed acceptable by preoperative duplex evaluation and intraoperative angioscopic evaluation, is our secondary bypass or rebypass conduit of choice. Although the need for graft revision is greater for arm vein bypass grafts, the primary assisted patency is 72% over 5 years.[22] We believe that vein grafts spliced together from lesser saphenous vein and remaining ipsilateral saphenous vein have patency equivalent to that of arm vein, but carry with them the added morbidity of distal incisions in a presently ischemic, previously operated limb. Use of arm vein as conduit also minimizes the number of venovenostomies. Utilization of the profunda femoris or endarterectomy of the superficial femoral artery to lessen the conduit length required for bypass is also a preferred technique. Others advocate repeat infragenicular bypass using prosthetic conduit aided by distal vein cuffs or arteriovenous fistula in these desperate circumstances.[23, 24] These are techniques we use rarely and only at last resort. Despite the optimal reports of others, our results in these patients have not been comparable to repeat bypass with autogenous vein.

SUMMARY

The best results in managing the failed infrainguinal vein graft are achieved by institution of protocols that maximize prevention. The first step is to discover and correct any problems in the bypass at the time of the initial surgery through rigorous assessment of the revascularization by measuring inflow pressure, inspecting the vein directly, performing valve lysis under angioscopic control, and using intraoperative ultrasound to evaluate the functioning graft and its outflow. An honest assessment of the likely long-term patency should be made at the conclusion of each case. Fruitless reexplorations can be avoided with the recognition that technical errors are unlikely using these techniques, and that the lack of other suitable conduit or bypass targets precludes further reasonable revascularization attempts. Unexpected early graft failures warrant screening for hypercoagulable states, and warrant immediate surgical reexploration with thorough evaluation of inflow, outflow, and conduit using repair or rebypass augmented with chronic systemic anticoagulation. Aggressive follow-up of graft function can detect patency-threatening lesions before thrombosis to ensure maintenance of optimal graft function. Patients whose grafts fail in the months after initial revascularization should be evaluated for the potential benefits of thrombolysis vs. surgery. Critical factors in treatment planning include the availability of autogenous vein for conduit and the condition of other distal arterial targets. Patient factors such as age, presence of diabetes, graft age, and presence of coronary artery disease can aid in the selection of graft and limb salvage techniques. Consideration of these risk factors will also permit choice of a bypass conduit that will optimize long-term survival and bilateral limb salvage among those patients who have severe, diffuse atherosclerosis of their lower extremities.

REFERENCES

1. Donaldson MC, Mannick JA, Whittemore AD: Femoral-distal bypass with in situ greater saphenous vein. Long-term results using the Mills valvulotome. *Ann Surg* 213:457–464, 1991.
2. Taylor LM Jr, Edwards JM, Porter JM: Present status of reversed vein bypass grafting: Five-year results of a modern series. *J Vasc Surg* 11:193–205, 1990.
3. Donaldson MC, Belkin M, Whittemore AD, et al: Impact of activated protein C resistance on general vascular surgical patients. *J Vasc Surg* 25:1054–1060, 1997.
4. Ascer E, Veith FJ, Morin L, et al: Components of outflow resistance and their correlation with graft patency in lower extremity arterial reconstructions. *J Vasc Surg* 1:817–28, 1984.

5. Schwartz LB, Belkin M, Donaldson MC, et al: Validation of a new and specific intraoperative measurement of vein graft resistance. *J Vasc Surg* 25:1033–1041, 1997.
6. Darling RC III, Chang BB, Shah DM, et al: Choice of peroneal or dorsalis pedis artery bypass for limb salvage. *Semin Vasc Surg* 10:17–22, 1997.
7. Bandyk DF, Johnson BL, Gupta AK, et al: Nature and management of duplex abnormalities encountered during infrainguinal vein bypass grafting. *J Vasc Surg* 24:430–436, 1996.
8. Miller A, Stonebridge PA, Tsoukas AI, et al: Angioscopically directed valvulotomy: A new valvulotome and technique. *J Vasc Surg* 13:813–820, 1991.
9. Gilbertson JJ, Walsh DB, Zwolak RM, et al: A blinded comparison of angiography, angioscopy, and duplex scanning in the intraoperative evaluation of the in situ saphenous vein bypass grafts. *J Vasc Surg* 15:121–127, 1992.
10. Miller A, Marcaccio EJ, Tannenbaum GA, et al: Comparison of angioscopy and angiography for monitoring infrainguinal bypass vein grafts: Results of a prospective randomized trial. *J Vasc Surg* 17:382–396, 1993.
11. Walsh DB, Zwolak RM, McDaniel MD, et al: Intragraft drug infusion as an adjunct to balloon catheter thrombectomy for salvage of thrombosed infragenicular vein grafts: A preliminary report. *J Vasc Surg* 11:753–759, 1990.
12. Robinson KD, Sato DT, Gregory RT, et al: Long-term outcome after early infrainguinal graft failure. *J Vasc Surg* 26:425–437, 1997.
13. Berkowitz HD, Kee JC: Occluded infrainguinal grafts: When to choose lytic therapy versus a new bypass graft. *Am J Surg* 170:136–139, 1995.
14. Nackman GB, Walsh DB, Fillinger MF, et al: Thrombolysis of occluded infrainguinal vein grafts: Predictors of outcome. *J Vasc Surg* 25:1023–1031, 1997.
15. Rose DA, Hertz SM, Eisenbud DE, et al: Endothelial cell adaption to chronic thrombosis. *Am J Surg* 174:210–213, 1997.
16. Stept LL, Flinn WR, McCarthy WJ III, et al: Technical defects as a cause of early graft failure after femorodistal bypass. *Arch Surg* 122:599–604, 1987.
17. DeFrang RD, Edwards JM, Moneta GL, et al: Repeat leg bypass after multiple prior bypass failures. *J Vasc Surg* 19:268–276, 1994.
18. Sanchez LA, Suggs WD, Marin ML, et al: Is percutaneous balloon angioplasty appropriate in the treatment of graft and anastomotic lesions responsible for failing vein bypasses? *Am J Surg* 168:97–101, 1994.
19. Houghton AD, Todd C, Pardy B, et al: Percutaneous angioplasty for infrainguinal graft-related stenoses. *Eur J Vasc Endovasc Surg* 14:380–385, 1997.
20. Sullivan TR Jr, Welch HJ, Iafrati MD, et al: Clinical results of common strategies used to revise infrainguinal vein grafts. *J Vasc Surg* 24:909–917, 1996.

21. Tarry WC, Walsh DB, Fillinger MF, et al: The fate of the contralateral leg following infrainguinal bypass. *J Vasc Surg*, 27:1039–1048, 1998.

22. Gentile AT, Lee RW, Moneta GL, et al: Results of bypass to the popliteal and tibial arteries with alternative sources of autogenous vein. *J Vasc Surg* 23:272–279, 1996.

23. Ascer E, Gennaro M, Pollina RM, et al: Complementary distal arteriovenous fistula and deep vein interposition: A five-year experience with a new technique to improve infrapopliteal prosthetic bypass patency. *J Vasc Surg* 24:134–143, 1996.

24. Raptis S, Miller JH: Influence of a vein cuff on polytetrafluoroethylene grafts for primary femoropopliteal bypass. *Br J Surg* 82:487–491, 1995.

CHAPTER 14

Subintimal (Extraluminal) Angioplasty of Femoropopliteal, Iliac, and Tibial Vessels

Amman Bolia, M.B.Ch.B., F.R.C.R.
Consultant Vascular Radiologist, Leicester Royal Infirmary, Leicester, England

Peter Bell, M.D., F.R.C.S.
Professor of Surgery, University of Leicester, Leicester, England

After the introduction of percutaneous endovascular techniques by Charles Dotter in 1964, and the introduction of the balloon catheter by Andreas Gruntzig, percutaneous transluminal angioplasty has become an accepted method for the treatment of peripheral vascular disease. The early treatment of atheromatous lesions was confined to short-segment stenosis[1] and occlusions because the equipment required to cross difficult lesions was not available. With time, new devices have been developed, and it is now possible to attempt more difficult lesions, longer occlusions, and disease in distal vessels.

However, the intraluminal approach has its limitations when treating very long occlusions of the femoropopliteal and tibial segments. The advent of subintimal angioplasty has allowed the treatment of long occlusions in those vessel segments[2] and also allows recanalization of long iliac occlusions using a combined ipsilateral and contralateral approach.

Subintimal recanalization is carried out using simple and conventional guidewires and catheters, and unlike other methods of treatment, does not require any expensive equipment or materials. It does not require extensive experience by the operator, and the technique offers a high success rate, a low complication rate, and is an inexpensive alternative to distal bypass surgery. It should

Advances in Vascular Surgery®, vol. 6
© 1998, Mosby, Inc.

195

therefore have wide application in the treatment of patients with peripheral vascular disease, particularly in those with chronic critical limb ischemia.

GENERAL

Our first patient was a 58-year-old man who was seen in January 1987 with a 19-month history of intermittent claudication at 100 yards. A diagnostic arteriogram demonstrated a 15-cm occlusion of the left popliteal artery. During attempted recanalization, the guidewire made an easy passage into the occlusion, and contrast injection confirmed extraluminal location of the catheter. The procedure was, however, continued and reentry was achieved in the distal popliteal artery. Subsequent balloon dilation of this extraluminal channel resulted in satisfactory flow through the angioplastied segment. A repeat angiogram 3 months after the recanalization demonstrated a normal-looking patent popliteal artery. The patient remained symptom free for 9.5 years until his death from other causes.

Subsequent to this accidental subintimal recanalization, further "accidents" followed and gradually we became aware that producing a channel using the extraluminal approach resulted in a satisfactory outcome, and increasingly it was noted that the cosmetic appearance of the resulting recanalized channel nearly always gave a very smooth appearance.

During those early days we postulated that this newly created channel was a more favorable one than an intraluminal channel because it was disease free and the extraluminal space was nearly always wider than the true lumen. Therefore if intimal hyperplasia developed, there would still be a large enough lumen for good flow to be maintained. In addition, the smooth disease-free channel allows laminar flow, which would favor minimal wall adhesion of platelets and therefore a low incidence of early reocclusion.

In view of the high primary success rates offered by the technique and improved long-term results, we now preferentially recanalize all occlusions using the extraluminal approach. The technique is mainly applicable in the femoropopliteal arteries and increasingly to the tibial and iliac arteries. Anecdotally, it has been applied in subclavian, brachial, and profunda artery occlusions as well.

INDICATIONS (FEMOROPOPLITEAL SEGMENT)

Very short occlusions (less than 3 cm), recent occlusions (less than 3–6 months old), and narrow vessels with extensive diffuse disease (less than 4 mm in diameter) are not usually dealt with by the extraluminal approach. However, if a dissection occurs during an attempted intraluminal approach, then subintimal recanalization is attempted.

Subintimal recanalization generally applies in the following situations:

1. Old Occlusions. It is difficult to tell how old an occlusion is. However, the length of the history, well-developed collaterals, and the presence of calcification all point to a long-standing occlusion and suitability for subintimal angioplasty.

2. Hard Occlusions. The hardness of an occlusion is determined by the feel imparted to the guidewire during an attempted re-canalization. The harder the occlusion feels, the longer it has been present and the more likely that dissection will be possible.

3. Long Occlusions. The longer the occlusion, the more difficult it is for the guidewire/catheter combination to remain intraluminal, and dissection is likely to occur.

4. Diffuse Disease. When there is an occlusion in an underlying diffusely diseased vessel, it is unlikely that the guidewire will negotiate the length of the occlusion while maintaining an intraluminal position. Dissection is likely to occur in these circumstances.

5. Previously Failed Intraluminal Approach. When there has been a previous attempt at recanalization and dissection has occurred, it is very unlikely that an intraluminal approach will be successful.

6. To Avoid a Large Collateral Entry. Occasionally a patient has a large collateral at the origin of an occlusion, and the resultant anatomy does not allow an intraluminal approach, because the guidewire will fail to engage into the true lumen of the main vessel but keep entering the collateral. In such situations, using the subintimal approach, one has to initiate a dissection in the main vessel, well above and in the opposite wall of the artery, away from the origin of the collateral. The dissection generally follows the route of the main vessel, avoiding the collateral.

7. Flush Occlusions. The technique of subintimal angioplasty allows flush occlusions of the superficial femoral artery without a stump to be dealt with.

TECHNIQUE

FEMOROPOPLITEAL OCCLUSIONS

An ipsilateral puncture of the common femoral artery is made for occlusions that begin from the origin of the superficial femoral artery. With the extraluminal approach, only a very small stump or no stump at all is needed. When there is a reasonable length of superficial femoral artery proximally, the puncture is usually made selectively into the superficial femoral artery itself. A 5F (van Andel type, Cook Limited, Letchworth, UK) predilating catheter is introduced and advanced to the origin of the occlusion.

Heparin (5,000 units) and tolazoline (12.5 mg) are injected before crossing the lesion. Tolazoline, a vasodilator, helps to dilate the distal vessels and reduce the possibility of spasm during the procedure. A straight floppy guidewire (3-cm floppy, 150-cm long, 0.035-inch diameter, Meadox, Dunstable, UK) is used to enter the occlusion (Fig 1,A). The tip of the wire is directed toward the arterial wall, taking care to avoid any large collaterals. Sometimes this requires either precurving the tip of the guidewire or using a preshaped catheter (Cobra). The wire/catheter combination is then advanced into the occlusion and, in the vast majority of cases, enters the path of least resistance, which is usually a dissection (Fig 1,B). Entry into the subintimal space is confirmed by injection of a small volume of dilute contrast medium (Fig 2). Once in the subintimal space the guidewire moves relatively freely, encountering little resistance. The straight guidewire is now replaced by a tapered-tip J wire (1.5-mm J, 150-cm long, 0.035- inch diameter, Meadox, UK). The length of the occlusion is traversed either by forward pressure on the J wire or by advancing the catheter with the J wire protruding from it. This combination usually allows crossing of most of the length of the occlusion. However, should there be any difficulty in traversing the length of the lesion because of its hardness or calcification, the J wire can be exchanged for any stiff guidewire. A stiff hydrophilic guidewire (Terumo, Tokyo, Japan) is our preferred choice.

When the catheter tip is 2–3 cm from the distal end of the occlusion, it is retracted by 2–3 cm and the J wire is manipulated to form a large loop (Fig 1,C). It is this large loop in the guidewire that enables the reentry into the true arterial lumen distally by use of forward pressure on the loop. The resistance to forward pressure will suddenly drop once the true lumen has been entered (Fig 1,D). Sometimes the dissection has to be extended further than the end of the occlusion to achieve reentry. This is usually of no con-

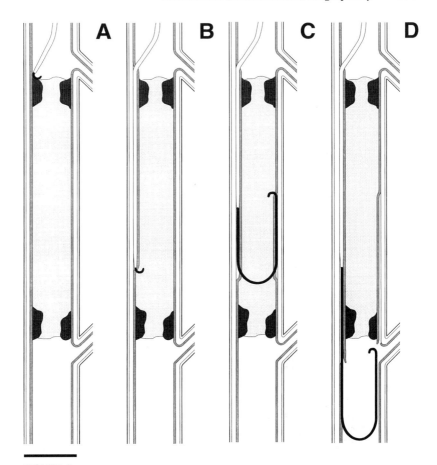

FIGURE 1.

Subintimal femoropopliteal recannalisation. **A,** the tip of the guidewire is directed towards the wall of the artery at the origin of the occlusion, opposite to the origin of a collateral. **B,** the catheter/wire combination enters the path of least resistance which is in a dissection **C,** the guidewire is manipulated to form a wide loop **D,** advancing the loop allows re-entry back into the lumen in the majority of the cases.

sequence to the patient unless some major collateral has been compromised without achieving reentry. To avoid this possibility, one should always avoid dissecting the origin of the most important and major collateral that reenters the artery beyond the occlusion. A collateral is frequently encountered at the midpopliteal level. Damage to this collateral must be avoided because it may be the last important collateral to the distal circulation. If there is an occlusion of the superficial femoral artery, the dissection can safely

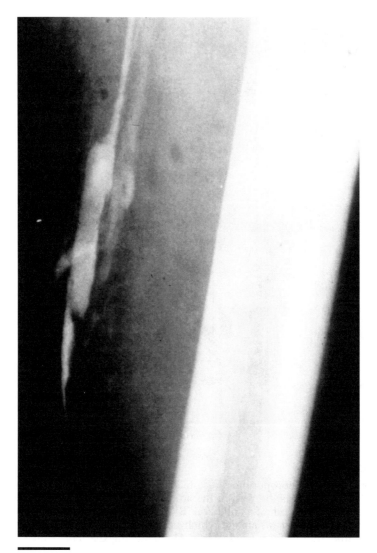

FIGURE 2.
Injection of contrast establishes that the subintimal space has been entered.

be extended up to the entry of this collateral into the popliteal artery. If luminal reentry has not been achieved by then, the procedure should be abandoned.

Once the lesion has been crossed, a 5F balloon catheter (usually 5 or 6 mm in diameter) is inflated throughout the entire length of the subintimal passage using approximately 10–12 atmospheres of pressure and 15-second inflations. If there is any residual stenosis of more than 30%, or if flow is impaired in any way, redilation is carried out using higher pressures until satisfactory flow is achieved. At the conclusion of the procedure, another dose of to-lazoline (12.5 mg) is given to achieve further vasodilation of the distal vessels to accommodate the improved flow from the recana-lized vessel (Fig 3).

Aspirin, if not contraindicated, is prescribed in patients who have had a successful recanalization; the usual dosage is 150 mg daily for 3 months. Oral anticoagulants are not used.

Special Situations

SMALL STUMP OR FLUSH OCCLUSION OF THE SUPERFICIAL FEMORAL ARTERY (SFA).—A high puncture is made in the ipsilateral common femo-ral artery to allow sufficient room for guidewire and/or catheter ma-neuvers. After needle insertion, a "roadmap" is obtained, prefer-ably with screening in an oblique plane to allow separation of the superficial femoral and profunda arteries.

A small curve is produced in an ordinary guidewire. This is achieved by running the soft tip of the guidewire between a thumb and index finger with some pressure exerted on the thumb to al-low the wire tip to curve. When there is a stump available, the tip of the guidewire can be manipulated into the stump, and further forward pressure on the guidewire will result in a dissection. Once the dissection has occurred, the van Andel predilating catheter can be introduced over the wire into the dissection. The straight wire is then substituted for a 1.5-mm J wire, and the rest of the proce-dure is as described above. If no stump is available and there is a flush SFA occlusion, then one has to rely on the guidewire tip to "catch" at the site of the SFA origin. Despite this catch, the soft end of the guidewire may not make an entry into a dissection. In such cases, the "hard" end of the wire with a slight curve imposed on it may initiate a dissection.

More recently we have been using a short 4F dilator passed into the common femoral artery, and through this "catheter" a curved hydrophilic guidewire (Terumo, Tokyo, Japan) allows a more guided manipulation toward the origin of the occluded SFA. Once again the hydrophilic guidewire "searches" for a catch at the ori-gin of the SFA, and once this catch is felt, the guidewire/catheter combination is gently manipulated into the origin of the occlusion. Once the occlusion is entered, the rest of the procedure is as de-scribed above.

FEMOROPOPLITEAL OCCLUSION IN THE PRESENCE OF A LARGE PROXIMAL COL-LATERAL.—This is a special situation where recanalization can only be achieved with a subintimal technique via an antegrade ap-

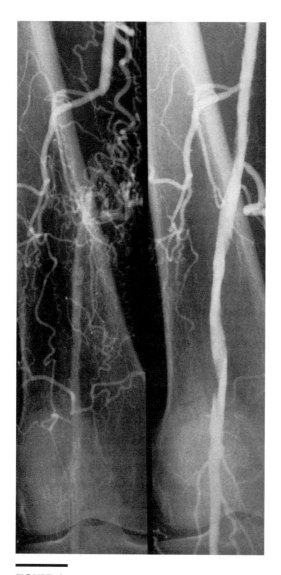

FIGURE 3.
Subintimal recanalization of femoropopliteal segment. The new channel has a typical spiral appearance.

proach. Alternatively, it can be done using a retrograde approach via a popliteal puncture.

When the proximal collateral is large and the occluded artery is without an apparent "stump" for the wire/catheter to engage, the guidewire will keep entering the collateral with some risk of damage to it. In such a situation, a dissection has to be initiated above the occlusion and well clear of the collateral. With the help of a curved catheter (Cobra shaped) and the "hard" end of the wire appropriately bent, and after a number of attempts, dissection will be achieved. Once the catheter is engaged in a dissection flap, the hard end of the wire is substituted for the J wire, and the rest of the procedure is as described above.

POPLITEAL OCCLUSION EXTENDING INTO THE TIBIAL VESSELS.—When patients are seen with a popliteal occlusion that extends into the tibial vessels, the initial symptoms are frequently those of critical ischemia, and therefore treatment is relatively urgent. Recanalization is planned so that a communication is created to as many of the patent tibial vessels as possible. This creates a situation where two important considerations come into play:

1. There is disparity in the size of the popliteal and tibial vessels, and therefore the procedure will require two different size balloon catheters (e.g., 5- and 3-mm diameter balloons).
2. When the guidewire is traversing the occlusion at the trifurcation, it comes across a choice of three possible entry points into the three tibial vessels.

The technique starts in a similar fashion to the femoropopliteal segment, but once the wire approaches the level of the trifurcation, the guidewire (usually an angled hydrophilic Terumo wire) is directed toward the vessel of interest. Hence, for example, if there is a good anterior tibial artery (AT) distally, the tip of the angled guidewire is directed toward where the anticipated origin of the AT might be. This is a "trial and error" situation because we do not know, while in the middle of an occlusion, where the AT origin might be. There is, however, usually a catch at the origin of the AT. At this point once a catch is felt, the tip of the wire is pushed into the AT with a predilating catheter (van Andel) following it. Once the wire has entered the occluded part of the AT, the wire is manipulated into a loop. Once again, as in the femoropopliteal segment, it is the loop in the wire that allows the dissection to be further advanced into the occlusion and allows subsequent reentry into the patent artery distally. A small balloon (e.g., 3 mm) is used to dilate the anterior tibial segment of the occlusion, and a larger balloon (e.g., 5 mm) is used for the rest of the popliteal segment.

If more than one good runoff vessel is seen distally, the aim is to recanalize in sequence all of them. For example, having created a communication into the AT first and satisfactorily recanalized the channel, the guidewire is then manipulated into the tibioperoneal trunk and then into the peroneal artery. Balloon dilation of the peroneal artery with a small (3 mm) balloon is carried out. Finally, the wire is manipulated into the posterior tibial artery, and subsequent dilation results in triple-vessel recanalization (Figs 4 and 5).

TIBIAL OCCLUSIONS

Short occlusions are usually crossed easily intraluminally, but subintimal recanalization is applicable for longer occlusions of 3 cm or more. The technique for crossing the lesion is basically similar to the approach used in the femoropopliteal occlusions except that we prefer to use a hydrophilic-angled guidewire (150-cm long, 0.035-inch diameter and angled, Terumo, Tokyo, Japan). Once again the aim is to form a loop in the guidewire as soon as the occlusion is entered. It is this loop that allows the dissection to be carried out throughout the length of the occlusion and also allows reentry into the lumen. Because the intima is much thinner as we go distally in the arterial tree, it is usually not difficult to reenter the true lumen in the distal tibial vessels. Balloon dilation is carried out in a similar fashion to the femoropopliteal segment. A 5F, 2-cm long, 3-mm diameter balloon is used to achieve dilatations using 10–12 atmospheres of pressure and 15-second inflations. Repeated inflations may be necessary if a satisfactory result has not been achieved in terms of improved flow or any residual stenoses (Fig 6).

Tolazoline (12.5 mg) is used before crossing the lesion, and a further dose is given after a successful recanalization. This helps to dilate the distal arteries and prevent spasm during the procedure. Should spasm occur despite the tolazoline, 100-μg boluses of intra-arterial nitroglycerine are administered (up to a maximum of 500 μg).

ILIAC OCCLUSIONS

A van Andel catheter (Cook Limited, Letchworth, UK) is introduced on the ipsilateral side up to the level of the distal part of the occlusion (Fig 7). The tip of an ordinary guidewire is curved by running the tip between the thumb and the index finger, with some pressure exerted on the thumb. The wire is then introduced

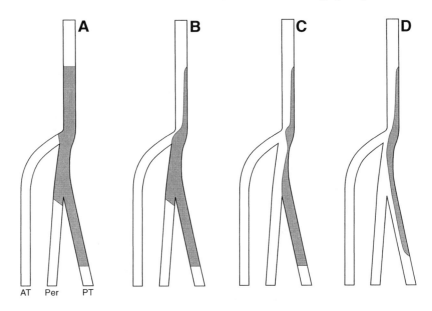

FIGURE 4.

Subintimal recannalisation of the popliteal tibial segments. *Abbreviations: AT,* anterior tibial artery; *Per,* peroneal artery; *PT,* posterior tibial artery. **A,** the popliteal occlusion extends into all three tibial arteries **B,** the occlusion into the anterior tibial artery has been recannalised first **C,** the recannalisation has been extended to the peroneal artery **D,** all three run off vessels have been recannalised **E,** the catheter position during a subintimal recannalisation **F,** the new recannalised subintimal lumen provides a smooth inner surface, as it is disease free.

through the van Andel catheter and the curved tip is directed towards the wall of the artery.

The wire is then advanced into the occlusion. Any resistance met during the attempted initiation of dissection is overcome by advancing the van Andel catheter to nearer the tip of the wire to strengthen the system and allow the force used on the wire to be directed to the wall of the artery. This invariably results in a dissection that is then further extended throughout the length of the occlusion with the help of a J wire.

An attempt is made to cross the occlusion through this dissection plane via the ipsilateral approach only. However, frequently reentry is difficult in such situations, and the tendency is for the catheter/guidewire to extend the dissection further toward the aorta. Attempts to reenter are abandoned once the dissection has extended into the aortic wall. Failure of reentry is probably caused by the thickness of the intima as the aorta is approached.

Subsequently, with the help of a sidewinder catheter (5F, 100-cm long, side winder II, Cordis UK Limited), the proximal part of the occlusion is approached via a crossover from the contralat-

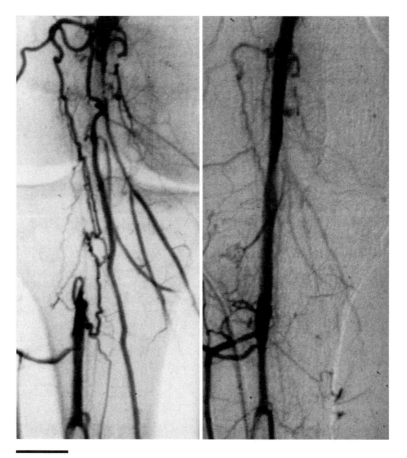

FIGURE 5.
A 6-cm popliteal occlusion before and after angioplasty.

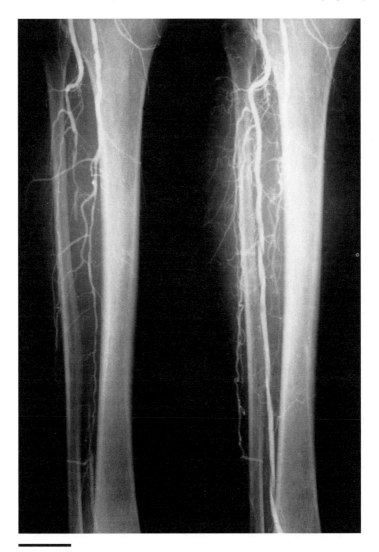

FIGURE 6.

A long occlusion of the anterior tibial artery has been reopened.

eral side. Once again a dissection is initiated in a similar fashion to the retrograde dissection. A curved tip hydrophilic guidewire (0.035-inch diameter, 3-cm floppy tip, 150-cm long, Terumo, Tokyo, Japan) is more helpful in creating a dissection from the crossover approach. Although the intima at this level may be thick, initiating a dissection is not a problem because any force directed at the ves-

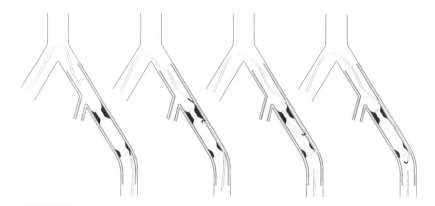

FIGURE 7.

The technique used for iliac recannalisation involves ipsilateral and contralateral subintimal dissections. **A,** a dissection is made retrogradely
through an ipsilateral puncture. An attempt is made to reenter but usually the dissection continues to extend upwards and failing to reenter. **B,**
a side-winder catheter introduced from the contralateral puncture is advanced to the proximal part of the occlusion and dissection initiated. **C,**
the dissection is extended with the use of a J wire. **D,** the J wire may meet
up with the dissection created retrogradely or may have to be converted
into a large loop, for the loop to reenter distal to the occlusion, the procedure being similar to the antegrade approach of femoropopliteal occlusions.

sel wall by the catheter/wire invariably allows the wire to take the
path of least resistance, which is in a dissection. Once the dissection has been initiated from the proximal part of the occlusion, it is
extended further distally. Because the proximal and the distal dissections are in the same plane, wire manipulations, usually with
the help of the hydrophilic wire, create a common channel. If the
common channel is not entered by simple wire manipulation, a
curved Terumo guidewire is manipulated into a wide loop. Advancing this loop helps to reenter the artery distally, as described
earlier. Once the guidewire has crossed the lesion, the sidewinder
catheter is substituted for a balloon catheter and the false channel
angioplastied via the crossover approach (Figs 7 and 8).

AFTERCARE

Generally after successful recanalization of an occluded segment,
the patient does not require any special care except in certain situations. In patients who have had recanalization of a long femoropopliteal or tibial occlusion, or have had a particularly difficult procedure, we recommend administering subcutaneous heparin, 5,000

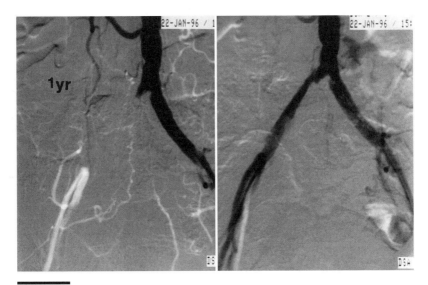

FIGURE 8.
Angiogram of right common iliac occlusion before and after recanalization.

units every 6 hours for a total of 4 doses, to prevent reocclusion of the angioplastied segment.

By encouraging peripheral vasodilatation in the treated leg, the resultant reduction in peripheral resistance improves flow through the angioplastied segment, which may help to maintain its patency during the early critical postprocedure phase. In most of our patients who have had recanalization of a long femoropopliteal or tibial occlusion, we apply a patch of glyceryl trinitrate to the affected leg; it delivers 5 mg of glyceryl trinitrate over 24 hours.

A high puncture is required to treat "flush" occlusions or occlusions with a very small stump of superficial femoral artery. Nursing staff must be made aware that a high puncture of the common femoral artery has been made, and the possibility of retroperitoneal haemorrhage must be considered if there are symptoms and signs of blood loss.

Unless contraindicated, all patients are prescribed 150 mg of aspirin daily for 3 months.

RESULTS

ILIAC ANGIOPLASTIES

Subintimal iliac recanalization has only been attempted by us on 35 occasions, with an immediate technical success rate of 70%. The

TABLE 1
Subintimal Angioplasty

Site	No. Pts	Technical Success	Hemodynamic Patency	
			12 mo	**36 mo**
Iliac	35	24 (70%)	90%	82%
Femoropopliteal	200	159 (80%)	73%	58%
Tibial	32	26 (81%)	50%	—

patency at 1 year for successful cases was 90% and at 3 years, 82% (Table 1).

FEMOROPOPLITEAL OCCLUSIONS
The results have been published elsewhere.[3] Briefly, during a 64-month period, 176 patients underwent 200 attempted subintimal angioplasty procedures for femoropopliteal occlusive disease. The primary technical success rate was 80% (159 of 200 patients) for a mean length of occlusion of 11 cm.

Technical success is defined as immediate restoration of the lumen of the artery without any stenosis greater than 30% and rapid reestablishment of flow. There were 14 minor complications (6.5%), mainly puncture site hematomas, and 2 major complications, 1 retroperitoneal and 1 scrotal haematoma, both of which required surgical evacuation. The hemodynamic patencies at 12 and 36 months for technically successful procedures were 73% and 58%, respectively (Fig 9).

TIBIAL OCCLUSIONS
The results have been published elsewhere. Of the 32 infrapopliteal artery occlusions in 28 critically ischemic limbs with a mean length of occlusion of 6 cm, the primary recanalization rate was 81% (26 of 32). There were 3 minor complications. The 1-year hemodynamic patency rate was 50%.[4–6]

IMPACT OF SUBINTIMAL ANGIOPLASTY ON CLINICAL PRACTICE
This technique has had a significant effect on the way we treat patients. It is very cost-effective; all that is required is a J wire, a van Andel catheter, and a 5F balloon catheter. The patient is usually admitted as a day case and does not incur any overnight costs in treatment, which obviously compares favorably with alternatives such

Symptomatic patency

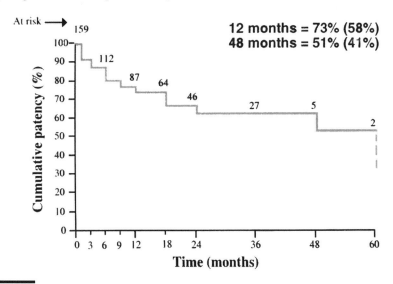

FIGURE 9.

The patency results of femoropopliteal subintimal angioplasty over a 4-year period.

as surgery. An additional benefit is the lack of mortality, which is significant in older patients having surgical treatment, particularly for critical ischemia. Our present policy is outlined below.

PATIENTS WITH CLAUDICATION

The patient arrives for a consultation, which is followed by an immediate duplex scan of the leg vessels. The patient is then seen again immediately after the scan and treatment options decided at the first visit. If the duplex scan suggests that femoropopliteal occlusion is present with good vessels below this, then subintimal angioplasty is attempted even for those with flush occlusions of the femoral artery. If this is successful, the claudication is abolished. If the angioplasty fails, then the patient is usually no worse off. No other treatment is provided unless there is further deterioration, in which case surgery may become necessary. Because of this technique, very few patients require surgery for claudication. In our unit this would amount to 10–15 patients per year who have severe claudication compared with angioplasty, which is used in 400–500 patients per year.

PATIENTS WITH CRITICAL ISCHAEMIA

The most significant impact on our workload has been in those patients with critical ischemia. When they are seen, a duplex scan is done first to determine whether there are distal runoff vessels below the occlusion. After this a subintimal angioplasty is attempted, and surgery follows if this is unsuccessful. The most recent results from our center[5] show that more than 49% of patients are now successfully dealt with by subintimal angioplasty, leaving about 30% needing reconstructive surgical treatment. The remainder are usually unfit for any form of treatment except amputation in some cases. This change has meant that our workload has diminished considerably, and we no longer have to spend significant amounts of time in the operating room dealing with patients who have crural disease. About one third of our patients are diabetic, and the technique is also successful in them.

The reason why subintimal angioplasty works is hard to be certain of but probably relates to the entirely new surface that is created which is not lined by endothelial cells and therefore does not have the tendency to stenose from intimal hyperplasia. A randomized study between this treatment and surgery has not been done yet but will probably be the next step. Presently, however, the mortality rate from surgery for patients with crural disease, who are often old and have multisystem failure, is such that by comparison, subintimal angioplasty is much safer with a much lower mortality rate to date.

CONCLUSION

Subintimal angioplasty of femoropopliteal and tibial artery occlusions can be performed with a high technical success rate and a low major complication rate. The possibility of subsequent bypass surgery is not compromised in patients with failed recanalization. The technique is safe, effective, and inexpensive in femoropopliteal occlusions. In infrapopliteal arteries, it offers a low-risk alternative to distal reconstructive surgery, particularly in elderly patients with critical limb ischemia. In a small number of patients there may be a suitable crural artery for a distal bypass, but the extent of ulceration, infection, edema, and quality of the skin may be such that surgery becomes impractical. Subintimal angioplasty may be a limb saver in such cases.[5]

In iliac occlusive disease, attempts at intraluminal recanalization frequently result in a dissection from the ipsilateral approach. With the help of the contralateral approach, the majority of dissections can be retrieved and facilitate a successful outcome. However, long-term patency results are, as yet, unavailable.

REFERENCES

1. Johnson KW: Femoral and popliteal arteries reanalysis: results of balloon angioplasty. *Radiology* 183:767–771, 1992.
2. Bolia A, Miles KA, Brennan J, et al: Percutaneous transluminal angioplasty of occlusions of the femoral and popliteal arteries by subintimal dissection. *Cardiovasc Int Radiol* 13:357–363, 1990.
3. London NJM, Srinivassan R, Naylor AR, et al: Subintimal angioplasty and femoropopliteal occlusion. Longterm results. *Eur J Vasc Surg* 8:148–155, 1994.
4. Bolia A, Sayers RD, Thompson MM, et al: Subintimal and intraluminal recanalization of occluded crural arteries by percutaneous balloon angioplasty. *Eur J Vasc Surg* 8:214–219, 1994.
5. Varty K, Nydahl S, Butterworth P, et al: Changes in the management of critical limb ischaemia. *Br J Surg* 83:953–956, 1996.
6. Nydahl S, Hartshorne T, Bell PRF, et al: Subintimal angioplasty of infrapopliteal occlusions in critically ischaemic limbs. *Eur J Vasc Endovasc Surg* 14:213–216, 1997.

CHAPTER 15

Creative Foot Salvage

John E. Connolly, D.P.M
Assistant Professor of Surgery (Podiatry), Dartmouth Medical School, Hanover, New Hampshire; Staff Podiatrist and Director, Podiatric Medical Education, Veterans Affairs Medical Center, White River Junction, Vermont

Martha D. McDaniel, M.D.
Associate Professor of Surgery, Dartmouth Medical School, Hanover, New Hampshire; Acting Chief, Surgical Service, Veterans Affairs Medical Center, White River Junction, Vermont

James S. Wrobel, M.S., D.P.M.
Adjunct Assistant Professor, Departments of Family and Community Medicine and Surgery (Podiatry), Dartmouth Medical School, Hanover, New Hampshire; Staff Podiatrist, Veterans Affairs Medical Center, White River Junction, Vermont

Kim M. Rozokat, C.O.T.A.
Certified Occupational Therapy Assistant, Veterans Affairs Medical Center, White River Junction, Vermont

S ome of the most challenging patients we are called upon to treat are those we have chosen to call "high risk": those with varying combinations of mechanical deformity, neuropathy, arterial insufficiency, and present or past ulceration of the foot. Typically, such patients followed in our multidisciplinary high-risk foot clinic are elderly and relatively sedentary, have a scanty social support structure at home, and have a panoply of comorbidities that contribute to high operative risk and compromised wound healing. At all times, our focus with these patients is to optimize their functional capacity, to minimize their dependence on hospital-based care, and to curb the trend toward institutionalization of these often infirm individuals.

The goals of our patients, in conjunction with their special medical circumstances, mandate that we push the limits of limb salvage and constantly search for successful ways to salvage a weight-bearing platform for them. It is our experience with this population that provides the background for the sometimes unconventional techniques we discuss in this chapter.

WHEN IS AN OPERATION REQUIRED?

When a patient is seen with a foot lesion, the primary question is whether it will heal without any intervention or with medical therapy alone. Predictors of healing of lesions involving only skin are numerous and include measures of skin blood flow and tissue oxygenation.[1] Foot radiographs should routinely be obtained to detect gas in the soft tissues or a foreign body, either of which would mandate operation. Prediction of wound healing becomes more complicated when a skin lesion tracks to bone, the patient is not systemically septic, and there is little or no local soft tissue involvement. The question in this case is whether the underlying bony lesion is osteitis or osteomyelitis. If the former, permanent resolution may be effected by medical means; if the latter, controversy abounds as to whether permanent resolution can ever be achieved by measures short of excision of the affected bone. Small case series[2] indicate that two thirds to three quarters of patients will escape amputation or recurrence during the year after treatment of osteomyelitis with administration of oral antibiotics. Higher certainty of cure[3] seems to result from treatment with 1–2 weeks of parenteral antibiotics in concert with debridement of infected bone.

Diagnosing pedal osteomyelitis, especially in diabetic patients, can be difficult. Arterial insufficiency or underlying osteoarthropathy of either the hypertrophic or atrophic type can confound the interpretation of diagnostic tests. Ninety-four percent of diabetic pedal osteomyelitis is contiguous with open ulceration.[4] Given this knowledge, application of Bayes' theorem[5] shows that probing to bone through the ulceration predicts the presence of osteomyelitis as well as MRI and/or scanning with technetium-99m or indium-111, or plain radiographs. Absence of osteomyelitis is best predicted by normal MRI. We restrict the use of percutaneous bone biopsy to situations in which patient preference for nonsurgical therapy is strong: both in this instance and when biopsy is done at the time of open bone debridement, culture results guide the subsequent choice of antibiotic.

A patient with marginally oxygenated feet may develop a trivial ischemic skin lesion or focal osteomyelitis. If it is clear that revascularization is not possible and that healing of the lesion or planned digital amputation site is unlikely, we believe that major amputation is not the only option in the context of many patients' goals. If the patient has a knowledgeable supporter at home who is able to recognize progression of infection; if sudden progression is improbable or would be unlikely to change the level of major amputation; and if the limb in question is important in maintaining independence (e.g., allows transfer after contralateral above-knee amputation and therefore allows the patient to remain at home), local wound care alone may allow the patient to retain the limb for a period that is substantial in the context of the patient's limited life expectancy.

PREOPERATIVE ASSESSMENT

It seems self-evident but is crucially important that no overall limb salvage plan be devised until the patient's systemic comorbidities, home situation, and goals are fully assessed.

SYSTEMIC EVALUATION

Systemic factors that may compromise wound healing are critical to recognize and optimize before operating in this marginal population. Special areas to consider are listed in Table 1.

HOME SITUATION

The likelihood of success of any limb salvage strategy is strongly dependent on the patient's home situation. Considerations include the individual's judgment; ability to comply with instructions; caretaker's eyesight and knowledge (and sometimes, strength) of significant others in the home or immediate neighborhood; the availability of, and payment mechanism for, a visiting nurse and other community services; ease with which the patient can return to the clinic for follow-up care; geography of the living space; and facilities for maintaining personal hygiene. Deficiencies in any of these may mandate institutionalization during the convalescent period. Investments in educating patients and their significant others concerning both the underlying medical problems and ways in which they can take charge of the outcome are richly rewarded.

PATIENT GOALS

Achieving a fully healed limb is normally the goal of treatment. However, an infirm patient with limited life expectancy may have important goals that are at odds with the considerable effort which may be required to achieve full healing. Arriving at a clear mutual understanding of the goals of treatment at the outset is critical to a successful interaction.

ASSESSMENT OF WOUND HEALING POTENTIAL AT THE PLANNED SURGICAL SITE

The systemic condition of the patient will often determine the correct choice of procedure if multiple options exist. For example, if peripheral edema is a prominent fixed feature, other determinants of wound healing potential such as tissue oxygenation will need

---

TABLE 1.
Factors to Assess Before Planning Foot Amputation

Factors	Comments
Systemic factors (myocardial infarction with or without congestive heart failure; anemia)	In chronically ill, sedentary, and/or neuropathic individuals, diminution of cardiac output or systemic oxygenation may be asymptomatic except for decrease in tissue oxygen delivery at foot level. The underlying condition should be recognized and treated.
Proteinuria and hypoalbuminemia in diabetics with nephropathy	The hypoalbuminemia associated with significant proteinuria can be associated with significant protein/calorie malnutrition and predispose lower extremites to edema formation. Antithrombin III is of low molecular weight and is lost through glomeruli in this condition. Systemic deficiency of antithrombin III may render a patient hypercoagulable.
Lower extremity edema	Underlying malnutrition, congestive heart failure, or deep venous thrombosis should be recognized and treated. Even if no underlying condition is found, edema ipsilateral to planned amputation should be minimized to promote wound healing. If simple extremity elevation fails, sequential compression devices may be useful.
Condition of skin adjacent to planned incision	If adjacent skin is dry, application of moisturizing agents may diminish risk of bacterial invasion. If skin adjacent to necrotic area is profoundly ischemic, delay of definitive foot procedure for several days after revascularization improves local wound healing.

(continued)

TABLE 1. (continued)

Factors	Comments
Condition of contralateral extremity	The contralateral extremity, if present, is the sole means of transfer and mobility for the postoperative period. If it functions well, expeditious return to the community is more likely. These limbs are prone to injury during the convalescent period from even minor chronic pressure. Decubitus injury to the heel is particularly devastating.
Nutritional status	Ideally, malnutrition would be remedied (serum albumin >3.0 g/dL and total lymphocyte count >1,500/μL) before definitive surgery. Although this is frequently impossible given the urgency imposed by infection, postoperative attention to nutritional status is critical in the promotion of wound healing. Supplementation of vitamins A and C, and of zinc may also be beneficial, particularly in steroid-dependent patients.
Prophylaxis against deep vein thrombosis	Enforced bed rest and various causes of hypercoagulability mandate careful attention to this detail.

to be optimal. If bacterial contamination is absent, tissue oxygenation at the planned surgical site is the single greatest determinant of wound healing. Noninvasive measurement of major arterial pressure at ankle level is notoriously unreliable in patients with diabetes and chronic renal failure because of arterial calcification. Overall, transcutaneous measurement of dermal oxygenation (T_cPO_2) appears to be the most accurate predictor of amputation site healing.[6] Therefore, except in the presence of abscess or advancing infection, revascularization (if needed) should precede any surgery in the foot.

AMPUTATION TECHNIQUES

Systemic issues having been addressed to the extent possible and wound healing potential having been optimized, it becomes time to devise a surgical plan that is most consistent with the patient's goals, is likely to allow complete wound healing, and will maximize function in the long-term as the foot and its supporting struc-

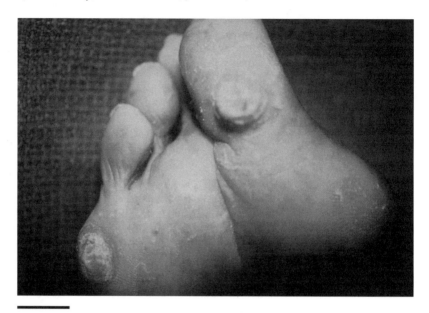

FIGURE 1.
Hallux abductovalgus (bunion) develops as a result of digital drift after proximal transphalangeal amputation of the second toe if prosthesis is not in place.

tures adjust to a new weight-bearing pattern. For many of the amputations described below, it is useful to clarify with the patient preoperatively that prosthetic and/or orthotic management will be a planned and important contribution to long-term success (defined as optimal function with minimal dependence on hospital-based care). What follows below are issues we have learned to consider, depending on the part of the foot that is involved. Although the level of detail of these discussions may seem extreme, we have found that both meticulous tissue handling and careful attention to such details are essential to achieving the desired results.

DIGITAL AMPUTATIONS
If single digital amputation is required, we prefer to perform this through the shaft of the proximal phalanx rather than to disarticulate at the metatarsophalangeal joint, to minimize subsequent drift of adjacent digits with hammertoe and/or hallux abductovalgus (bunion) formation (Fig 1). After amputation even at the transphalangeal level of the second toe, the problem of drift is so pronounced and so potentially dangerous that we frequently fabricate a prosthesis out of fast-curing moldable compound for daily

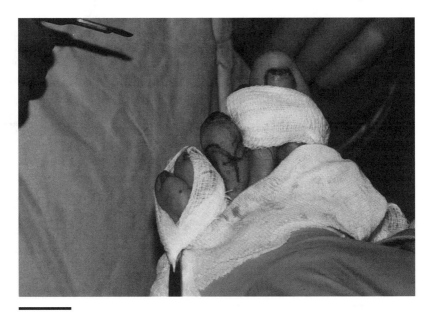

FIGURE 2.

Diagram of skin incision recommended for single proximal transphalangeal toe amputation.

wear as soon as the wound is healed. A dorsal-to-plantar fishmouth incision (Fig 2) allows for dependent drainage and rapid wound healing after transphalangeal amputation. In our experience, rotation of the same incision so that the fishmouth is oriented in the medial-lateral direction is associated with traction, dehiscence, and collection of serum and blood at the amputation site. This is particularly a problem after amputation of the fifth digit in a patient with predilection for equinus deformity. If the issue of soft tissue coverage or extensive osteomyelitis of the proximal phalanx mandates amputation of the entire digit, reasonable efforts should be made to preserve the metatarsal head, thereby preserving the metatarsal parabola. When disarticulation is performed, it has been our practice to denude the articular cartilage from the metatarsal head with a rongeur or a rasp. Although it has been suggested that the articular cap may act as a barrier against infection, we believe that without synovial fluid to provide nutrients to the hyaline cartilage, it will necrose and become a possible nidus for infection.

The "intrinsic-minus" foot type (high medial arch with significant hammertoe deformity and extensor tendon bowing) characteristic of the diabetic typically leads to lesions on the dorsal surface

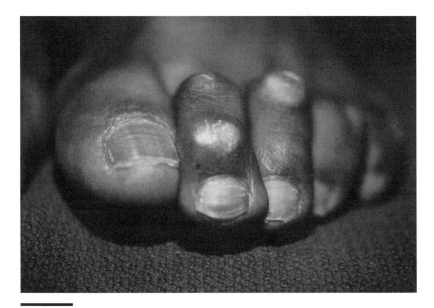

FIGURE 3.
The dorsal surface of hammertoes is particularly vulnerable to shoe-induced lesions in the intrinsic-minus foot type. (Courtesy of Anne Sonoga, D.P.M.)

of multiple toes from inappropriate shoes (Fig 3). In this and other situations in which amputation of more than one digit is required to achieve soft tissue coverage, we strongly consider simultaneous performance of proximal transphalangeal amputation of all five toes, on the grounds that this reduces the likelihood of subsequent infections in the remaining exposed digits. Additionally, patients returning for a second episode of digital amputation of the same foot will be considered for a pandigital amputation. The concept of a "digital parabola" has not been as significant as identifying the mechanism of injury leading to amputation of the digit. If the mechanism is not reversible, such as with neuropathy or compliance issues, our threshold is lowered. With the intrinsic-minus foot, the hyperextension at the metatarsophalangeal joint causes migration of the amputation sites dorsally to the non–weight-bearing surface (Fig 4). Release of the long extensor tendon in the course of transphalangeal amputation markedly reduces the retrograde pressure on the corresponding metatarsal head. Regardless, touchdown weight-bearing can be resumed much more rapidly after transphalangeal than after transmetatarsal amputation, and patient return to the community is therefore more rapid. In addition,

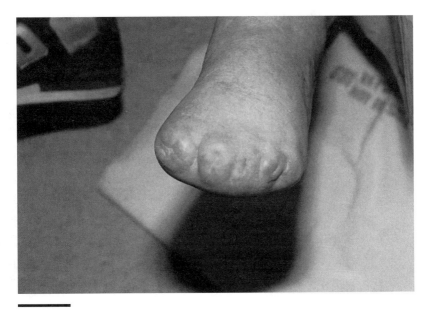

FIGURE 4.

Healed foot after transphalangeal amputation of all five toes. Both transversely and vertically oriented skin incisions were used, but the incisions are well away from the weight-bearing surface of the foot.

this approach preserves important and scarce durable tissue for subsequent transfer if a second forefoot procedure becomes necessary. If multiple transphalangeal amputations are performed simultaneously, an alternating pattern of vertical and horizontal incisions may be required to diminish skin tension at the time of closure.

Hallux amputation is regarded by some as unwise because of the role of the hallux in maintaining balance.[7] Hallux preservation is generally desirable, and extra effort to preserve as much length as possible will be rewarded. While it is true that the hallux is central to allowing normal propulsive (heel-toe) gait, patients with advanced neuropathy and proprioceptive loss frequently exhibit an apropulsive gait pattern that relies much less heavily on the hallux. Therefore, if hallux amputation through the proximal phalangeal shaft is required to achieve a healed wound in this population, poor balance and transfer lesions (subsequent ulcerations over new pressure points) have not been prominent problems in our experience. Incisional design and placement are also important in achieving a successful, long-term result after hallux amputation. In contrast to the optimal incisional placement and design for

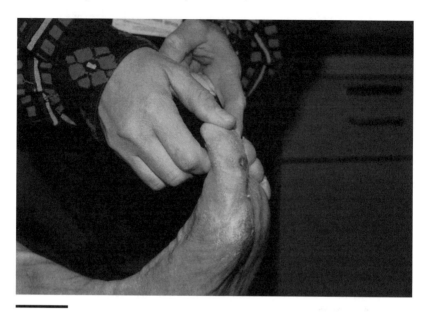

FIGURE 5.

Hallux rigidus at maximum extension. The primary skin lesion is plantar to the proximal phalanx, with substantial callus beneath the first metatarsal head.

transphalangeal amputation of the lesser toes, wound healing and soft tissue coverage on the weight-bearing surface are optimized by the use of a terminal Syme incision (long plantar flap so that the suture line is relatively dorsal) when working with the hallux.

Another special consideration in hallux amputation is maintaining the insertion of the flexor hallucis brevis muscle at the base of the proximal phalanx. This tendon contains the sesamoid apparatus within its substance. As long as the tendon remains intact, the sesamoids move under the first metatarsal head and effectively lengthen the first ray in the propulsive phase of normal gait. If the two pea-sized sesamoid bones become static, however, they scar in place under the first metatarsal head and effectively become an exostosis, leading to increased pressure and ulceration. Therefore, if disarticulation at the first metatarsophalangeal joint is required, we strongly recommend simultaneous removal of the sesamoids.

In hallux limitus, the proximal phalanx is relatively plantarly subluxed on the first metatarsal head, and therefore cannot glide dorsally over the metatarsal head during the pushoff phase of propulsive gait. This common clinical scenario (Fig 5) leads to ulceration of the plantar surface of the first proximal phalanx or first

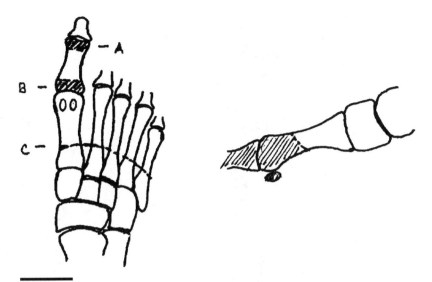

FIGURE 6.

Left-hand drawing shows dorsal view of diverse forefoot procedures. A: bone to be resected (shaded) in hallux interphalangeal arthroplasty; B: bone to be resected in metatarsal-phalangeal arthroplasty; C: correct metatarsal parabola for full transmetatarsal amputation. Right-hand drawing: lateral view showing bone and sesamoids to be resected in full transmetatarsal amputation.

metatarsal head, largely resulting from the shear force generated as the patient compensates by pivoting on the forefoot. The appropriate salvage procedure for a first ray in the former situation is interphalangeal joint arthroplasty of the hallux; in the latter situation, hemiphalangectomy of the proximal phalangeal base.[8] If the base of the first ray is resected, the sesamoids should be removed or freed to migrate proximally (Fig 6).

RAY AMPUTATIONS

It goes without saying that ray amputations produce more deformity than digital amputations. With the loss of one metatarsal head, the general fear is that the metatarsal arch of the foot will be destroyed and the patient will therefore become susceptible to transfer lesions. For this reason, ray amputations are uncommonly performed in general practice.

Before discussing issues specific to ray amputation, it is useful to clarify the concept of the metatarsal parabola (Fig 6).[9] The metatarsal heads form a parabolic curve that promotes uniform lateral-to-medial loading of the forefoot in normal walking. Uniform dis-

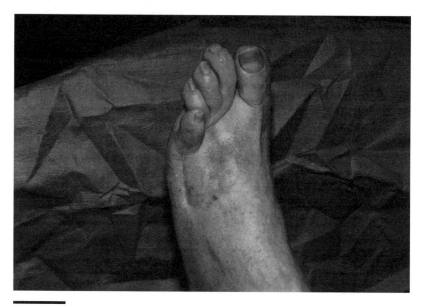

FIGURE 7.
Dorsal contracture of the digit after fifth metatarsal head resection.

persion of forces across the ball of the foot minimizes areas of focal pressure and ulceration. Detailed knowledge of midfoot anatomy, as well as consideration of the special characteristics of the high-risk foot population, helps to inform decisions concerning the advisability of ray amputations. The mechanics and anatomy of the fifth, first, and second/third/fourth rays are different from each other. For example, the fifth ray has a sizable dorsal excursion. The practical implication is that once the metatarsal head has been resected, this ray no longer bears weight and can therefore be safely resected as far proximally as necessary to achieve a tension-free wound closure with no additional adverse long-term consequences. The risk of transfer lesions with a fifth ray resection is minimal. The most common sequela of isolated fifth metatarsal head resection is dorsal contracture of the digit (Fig 7), although with provision of appropriate shoes this is rarely an important clinical problem.

The first ray, in contrast, is a key element in normal weight-bearing in that it carries half of the force exerted through the foot. If disarticulation of the hallux is required, it is wise not only to resect sesamoids as discussed above, but to resect the metatarsal head as extensively as is necessary (up to one fourth of the metatarsal length) to allow tension-free wound closure and to place more durable tissue on the weight-bearing surface. The first metatarsal should be resected from the medial cortex distally toward the second metatarsal head, in line with the desired metatarsal parabola. After distal first metatarsal resection, the relative dorsal excursion of the first metatarsal allows gradual loading of the lateral metatarsals. The lost weight-bearing function of the first ray can be compensated for by postoperative orthotic support of the arch with a generous cradling medial flange. This distributes through the medial arch weight-bearing forces that would otherwise be borne primarily by the second metatarsal head. This is particularly critical in the rare instance when an isolated first ray resection is considered.

As more of the first metatarsal is resected (and the lever arm of the first ray shortens), weight transfer to the second metatarsal becomes more abrupt. Resulting peak pressures can exceed the capacity of orthotic management to compensate. To prevent second metatarsal stress fracture (Fig 8) or ulceration, surgical remodeling with a partial second metatarsal resection to achieve a smooth parabolic curve across the metatarsal heads is required. Deossification of the second digit with preservation of its skin can also provide a well-vascularized, sensate flap to aid in closure of the wound at the site of first metatarsal resection.

Although uncommonly necessary, resection of a single central ray may be indicated in a patient with normal propulsive gait and good healing potential. We discourage isolated metatarsal head resection in the central rays, because transfer lesions occur more commonly here than after first or fifth metatarsal head resection. Achieving successful long-term foot function after resection of a central ray requires that the foot be narrowed so that weight distribution is even across the remaining metatarsal heads. In view of the restrictive nature of the deep transverse intermetatarsal ligaments connecting the second, third, and fourth rays, and the stability of the ligament complex and articulations at the metatarsal-cuneiform and metatarsal-cuboid joints, this is a unique challenge. If the metatarsals adjacent to the resected ray cannot mobilize to fill the void, they will carry an increased load and cause ulceration. Eighty percent resection of the affected ray seems to allow the adjacent metatarsal heads to migrate sufficiently to maintain midfoot stability and reconstitute an effective metatarsal parabola (Fig 9). We caution against complete resection of a central ray. Disruption of the Lis Franc ligament complex at the tarso-metatarsal junction leads to hypermobility and instability of the remaining central rays.

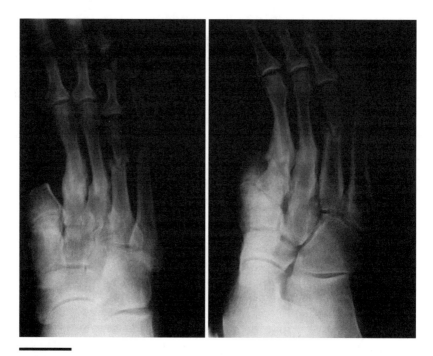

FIGURE 8.
Complete resection of the first ray alone puts excessive force on the lateral rays, sometimes leading to fracture. (Courtesy of Craig Christenson, D.P.M.)

In our patient population this can easily precipitate a most unwelcome midfoot Charcot deformity.

FULL TRANSMETATARSAL AMPUTATION
When forefoot necrosis is extensive, full transmetatarsal amputation frequently is the choice most consistent with long-term durability. Again, considerations of anatomy and normal gait are important in achieving a satisfactory long-term result.[10] Although the metatarsal heads are removed during this procedure, achieving a smooth metatarsal parabola with the residual metatarsal shafts is still important in avoiding future ulceration (Fig 10). The second metatarsal-cuneiform joint is deceptively distal. We therefore advise commencing the procedure on the medial side, because the curve is easier to predict accurately if the second metatarsal is resected at a point sufficiently distal to the metatarsal-cunneiform joint early during the procedure.

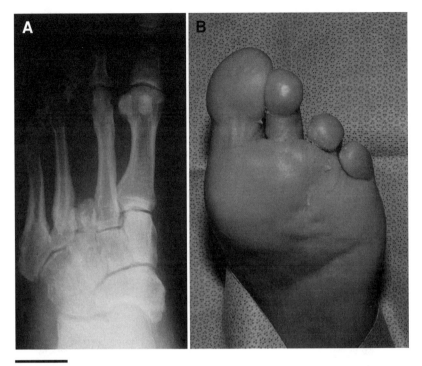

FIGURE 9.
Isolated resection of the majority of the third ray. **A,** radiograph showing extent of ray resection. **B,** plantar view of healed foot. Note smooth parabola described by the remaining metatarsal heads, as well as their distribution.

Typically, transmetatarsal amputation is planned with long plantar and short dorsal skin flaps. However, this general plan frequently requires creative modification to deal with areas of tissue loss, particularly plantar ulcers beneath the metatarsal heads. The correct plan will be determined by the amount of healthy plantar tissue available for closure. If tissue is plentiful, we resect the wound and its hypertrophic fibrous rim. If tissue is at a premium, we have found it acceptable to debride the wound and use the ulcer as a point of egress for a wick or Kritter drain (see below). If the latter course is indicated, the defect will not be on a weight-bearing surface once the plantar flap has been rotated to cover the metatarsal shafts. The fundamental underlying principle is that scar or fragile skin on a weight-bearing surface is susceptible to breakdown resulting from the shear forces of gait.

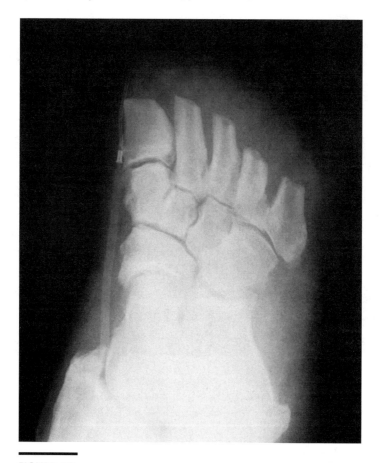

FIGURE 10.

A smooth parabola is described by the residual metatarsals after transmetatarsal amputation. A Kritter drain is in place.

Myriad technical issues are important in achieving a successful transmetatarsal amputation.[11] Minimization both of tissue trauma and dessication during the procedure are critical. Use of the power saw allows for better osseous remodeling. Bone should be divided perpendicular to the longitudinal axis of the metatarsal shaft. In practice, because of the normal angulation of the metatarsals, this corresponds to an angled cut of 20 degrees or more (proximal plantar to distal dorsal) in relation to the weight-bearing surface. It is also advisable to rasp the plantar cortex into a smooth curve.

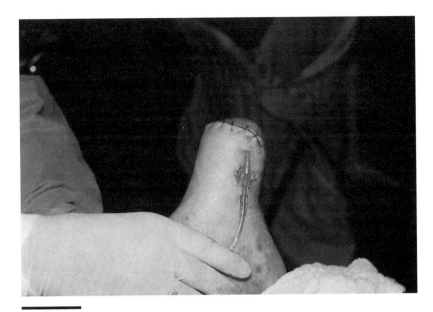

FIGURE 11.
Kritter drain in place after transmetatarsal amputation.

Use of the ingress/egress antibiotic infusion and drainage system as described by Kritter[12] has seemed to allow improved limb salvage in marginal situations. This system involves infusion of concentrated gentamicin solution (80 mg/L normal saline) through a 16-gauge angiocatheter into the transmetatarsal amputation site at the rate of 1 L per 24 hours for the first 48–72 hours after the operation, allowing egress of the fluid through the loosely closed incision (Fig 11). No dressing changes are made during this period except to apply absorbent bandage over the operative dressing. At this concentration, gentamicin has a much broader spectrum than when administered intravenously. The technique allows primary closure of a minimally infected wound. Diminution of hematoma formation is a possible additional benefit. Beveling the catheter before insertion, suturing the catheter to the skin, using an infusion pump, and slightly withdrawing the catheter if flow is impeded will help the infusion go smoothly.

A balance of strength between the muscle compartments is critical if any semblance of normal gait is to be preserved, in that this helps the foot to clear the ground as the limb swings forward. Resection of the phalanges and metatarsal heads necessitates division of the extensor hallucis and digitorum. This leaves the tibialis anterior (attached to the base of the first metatarsal-cuneiform joint) and the peroneus brevis (attached to the base of the fifth metatarsal) as the major dorsiflexors of the ankle. If imbalance between these opposing muscle groups develops, either because of resection of the muscular insertion site (base of the first or fifth metatarsal) or because of myopathy, equinovarus deformity develops at the ankle. Resulting pressure points may eventually lead to stump breakdown. Failure from this cause may be averted by percutaneous tendoachilles lengthening. This allows ankle dorsiflexion and shortens stride length, which in turn reduces forces applied to the foot.

Panmetatarsal head resection is sometimes proposed as a solution to refractory plantar ulceration. Most commonly performed in patients with rheumatoid arthritis, it has recently enjoyed some acceptance in the high-risk foot population.[13] Because it preserves the long extensors, long flexors, lumbricals, interossei, and the plantar fascia, it is believed that foot function is minimally affected; however, this has not been rigorously assessed. Dorsal digital drift is commonly seen after this procedure, but has not seemed to present a clinically significant problem in the rheumatoid population. In short, panmetatarsal head resection seems to have a sound safety profile in certain circumstances, but its role in the treatment of high-risk dysvascular feet is not well defined.

REARFOOT AMPUTATIONS

Amputations closer to the rearfoot than the conventional transmetatarsal amputation (Lis Franc, Chopart and Syme) have occasionally been advocated.[14] Anatomical considerations help explain why we regard these as operations of last resort. We would suggest that only a narrow spectrum of patients may benefit from such procedures as opposed to a below-knee amputation. Considerations in assessing patients for hindfoot amputations include use of the limb for transfer if this is the sole limb; significance of increased energy expenditure if a below-knee amputation is done instead, although this is generally a small variation; and the potential for a durable result (patient compliance, arterial supply, tissue quality). In short, we recommend whatever amputation patients will tolerate in the short-term and long-term while preserving their preoperative function as much as possible.

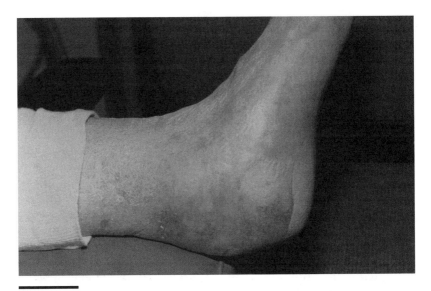

FIGURE 12.

Partial calcanectomy can result in durable limb salvage with good patient function. This partial calcanectomy was performed more than 40 years before the photograph was taken.

MANAGEMENT OF HEEL LESIONS

The heel is suseptible to deep infections, because the local adipose tissue is poorly vascularized and the area is subjected to high pressures both at rest and during ambulation. A clinically benign appearance of the skin at this level may fail to reflect the extent of underlying infection or necrosis. Appropriate management of heel wounds is difficult to choose. On one hand, because of the thinness of overlying tissue and because of the difficulty in delivering circulating antibiotics, aggressive debridement of heel wounds is risky. On the other hand, insufficient debridement may promote progression to calcaneal osteomyelitis. However these wounds are managed, complete relief of pressure is mandatory (see below).

If calcaneal osteomyelitis should be present subjacent to a heel ulcer, and the patient is compliant and has good systemic healing potential, partial calcanectomy may provide a durable solution short of major amputation (Fig 12). Excision of the affected portion of the calcaneus eradicates the bone infection and allows tension-free closure with excision of the wound. Once healed, it allows emergent ambulation without a prosthesis. For normal walking, the patient is provided with a custom molded shoe and usually a patellar tendon brace.

WOUND MANAGEMENT

Medical management of open wounds is often an important element in achieving final success in salvaging limbs. The basic goals of wound care are to provide an optimally moist environment, provide protection from pressure, provide substrates for healing, and prevent superinfection. Ideally, a wound management system will also be easy to use and inexpensive.

Clinical appearance of a wound provides clues of the degree to which current treatment meets the basic goals described above. If wound margins are free from maceration, the wound is not too moist; if wound margins are free from hyperkeratosis, pressure relief is adequate; if granulation is occurring, oxygen supply and systemic nutrition are adequate; if necrotic tissue and debris are absent, superinfection is improbable.

The full spectrum of wound management involves cleansing, debridement, dressing, and adjunctive therapies. Traditionally, various antiseptics (e.g., 10% povidone-iodine, chlorhexidine, Dakins solution, acetic acid solution, and hydrogen peroxide) have been used to clean wounds. These agents are cytotoxic and delay wound healing by 7% to 15%.[15] Agency for Health Care Policy and Research (AHCPR) guidelines[16] advise against their use except in preparation of surgical sites. As an alternative, wounds can safely be irrigated with normal saline solution at 4–15 psi using a 30-mL syringe and a 16-gauge angiocatheter.[16]

Necrotic tissue should always be debrided to a level where capillary bleeding occurs, except when the lesion is on the heel, lacks signs of infection, and has a stable eschar. If the usual sharp method of debridement is inadvisable because of a patient's limited ability to heal, selective enzymatic debridement (e.g., Elase, Accuzyme) for several days may be appropriate. Mechanical debridement using moistened gauze or sterile scrub brushes may be used when light films cover the wound. Dressings that are truly applied damp and removed dry normally provide sufficient ongoing debridement. Patients and their caretakers may require reassurance that they need not apply such a dressing dripping wet or soak it to take it off.

Selection of specific primary and secondary dressings should be based upon the clinical appearance of the wound. Alteration in appropriate dressing choice during the course of wound healing is common and does not reflect an error in the primary choice of dressing type. Superficial wounds can be covered with protective translucent films (e.g., OpSite, Tegaderm), which need to be changed every 2–3 days. Granulating nondraining wounds can be treated with hydrocolloids (e.g., Duo-derm, Restore), which can stay in place for 1–5 days at a time. Granulating wounds with minimal drainage can be treated with hydrogels (e.g., Normlgel, Aquasorb); these are more easily contoured than hydrocolloids but need to be changed every 1–3 days. Heavily draining wounds can be managed with foams (e.g., Mitraflex, Flexzan) and alginates (e.g., Sorbsan, Dermasorb); appropriate frequency of dressing changes depends on the amount of drainage but should not exceed 2–3 days. Classic saline damp to dry dressings are used for limited periods to accomplish mechanical debridement. Regardless of the dressing regimen chosen, wounds will not heal if they are subjected to pressure exceeding the local blood flow. Complete relief of pressure is of paramount importance.

Adjunctive therapies may prove useful for patients with inadequate blood supply and who are not candidates for revascularization. Systemic hyperbaric oxygen, periulcer ultrasound, electrical stimulation of the spinal cord, and platelet-derived wound healing factors all have been shown to increase wound healing if these modalities are available. We have found topical phenytoin (e.g., Dilantin) can be used to initiate granulation in wounds that fail to respond to other dressing techniques. The drug is usually applied by breaking a standard 100-mg capsule and lightly dusting the wound, which is then covered with saline-dampened gauze or hydrogel and gauze.

SHOES AND ORTHOTIC DEVICES

Virtually all foot lesions in this population are caused by focal pressure that exceeds the capacity of the tissues to remain intact. The first line of treatment for locally high pressures is to find or make accommodative footwear, rather than to change the contour of the foot. Physical examination, including identification of ulcers or preulcerative lesions, calluses, bony protuberances, and observation of the patient's gait pattern, will help determine specifically appropriate accommodations.

Fewer than 40% of individuals can actually find "off-the-shelf" shoes that fit correctly. Ill-fitting shoes can induce malalignment and promote abnormal foot motions, which result in feet that are pushed, pressed, and distorted. Malalignment over time changes muscle lever arms and may potentially alter the entire skeletal structure of the body.

Custom orthopedic ("extra-depth") shoes are fabricated over a measured last to allow for proper length (1/2 inch from the longest toe), width, contour, and heel counter of the patient's foot. These lightweight shoes can be made with special characteristics such as a high, soft toe box, extra-depth heel cups, soft leather uppers, and Velcro closures. With special attention to orthotic adjuncts, this type of shoe can accommodate most foot types. However, feet that are severely malaligned and unstable (e.g., those with the Charcot deformity, severe bunions, or severe, rigid hammertoes) may require even more customized footwear, such as a molded shoe. This is made from a plaster cast of the foot and is custom fabricated to account for foot contours and biomechanics. Many custom features are available. Built-in rocker soles and metatarsal bars aid in minimizing peak pressures caused by restricted joint motions. The orthotic insert can be modified to reduce pressure at sensitive calloused areas. Other features include high and wide toe boxes, counter supports to medial and lateral columns, custom shock- and shear-reducing inserts, and flared soles for increased stability while walking.

Interim footwear may be needed by patients who can walk or bear limited amounts of weight, but who have bulky dressings or temporary special needs. Rubber-soled sandals with lightweight, permeable uppers that close with Velcro can be used with custom orthotics to protect areas of the forefoot. The wedge or Carville rocker sole allows for off-loading of the distal forefoot. Weight-bearing pressure can be redistributed from the foot to the whole lower leg by using commercially available walking splints that immobilize the ankle. Full rocker soles in this setting allow for forward propulsion. However, this technique significantly alters gait and may be unwise to use in unsteady patients.

Special devices can meet the needs of nonambulatory patients for pressure relief. Calf-high foam boots have easily moveable foam inserts that can be positioned to minimize pressure when patients are in their usual resting position. These are ideal for night use or for bedridden patients. Alternatively, the heel of a wheelchair-bound patient can be completely suspended using a Linard splint, which has metal supports and sheepskin liners.

CONCLUSION

Salvage of a weight-bearing platform has important consequences for the fragile population of patients with mechanical deformity, neuropathy, arterial insufficiency, and present or past ulceration of the foot. Synthesis of knowledge about pedal anatomy, determinants of wound healing, the living situation and goals of a fragile patient, and the expected effect of weight-bearing on the ultimate shape and function of the foot after specific procedures permits sound decision making when such a patient requires pedal amputation to regain skin integrity. Careful choice of procedure, its meticulous execution, orthotic expertise, and long-term commitment to patient follow-up can be combined to maximize function in these difficult-to-treat patients.

REFERENCES

1. Ballard JL, Eke CC, Bunt TJ, et al: A prospective evaluation of transcutaneous oxygen measurements in the management of diabetic foot problems. *J Vasc Surg* 22:485–492, 1995.
2. Nix DE, Cumbo TJ, Kuritsky P, et al: Oral ciprofloxacin in the treatment of serious soft tissue and bone infection: Efficacy, safety, and pharmacokinetics. *Am J Med* 82(Suppl 4A):146–153, 1987.
3. Lipsky BA: Osteomyelitis of the foot in diabetic patients. *Clin Infect Dis* 25:1318–1326, 1997.
4. Bamberger DM, Daus GP, Gerding DN: Osteomyelitis in the feet of diabetic patients. *Am J Med* 83:653–660, 1987.
5. Wrobel JS, Connolly JE: Making the diagnosis of osteomyelitis: The role of prevalence. *J Am Podiatr Med Assoc* 88(7): in press.
6. Padberg FT, Back TL, Thompson PN, et al: Transcutaneous oxygen (T_cPO_2) estimates probablity of healing in the ischemic extremity. *J Surg Res* 60:365–369, 1996.
7. Lavery LA, Lavery DC, Quebedeax-Farnham TL: Increased foot pressures after great toe amputation in diabetes. *Diabetes Care* 18:1460–1462, 1995.
8. Rosenblum BI, Chrzan JS, Giurini JM, et al: Preventing loss of the great toe with the hallux interphalangeal joint arthroplasty. *J Foot Ankle Surg* 33:557–560, 1994.
9. Bauer G: Foot reconstruction after ablative debridement for severe diabetic foot infection. *Clin Podiatr Med Surg* 7:509–521, 1990.
10. Chrzan JS, Giurini JM, Hurchik JM: A biomechanical model for the transmetatarsal amputation. *J Am Podiatr Med Assoc* 83:82–86, 1993.
11. McKittrick LS, McKittrick JB, Risley TS: Transmetatarsal amputation for infection or gangrene in patients with diabetes mellitus. *Ann Surg* 130:826–842, 1949.
12. Kritter AE: A technique for salvage of the infected diabetic gangrenous foot. *Orthop Clin North Am* 4:21–30, 1973.
13. Guirini JM, Basile P, Chrzan JS, et al: Panmetatarsal head resection: A viable alternative to the transmetatarsal amputation. *J Am Podiatr Med Assoc* 83:101–107, 1993.

14. Chang BB, Bock DEM, Jacobs RL, et al: Increased limb salvage by the use of unconventional foot amputations. *J Vasc Surg* 19:341–349, 1994.

15. Alvarez OM: Pharmacological and environmental modulation of wound healing, in Vitto J, Parejda AJ (eds): *Connective Tissue Disease, Molecular Pathology of the Extracellular Matrix*. New York, Marcell Dekker, 1987, p 367–364.

16. Bergstrom N, Bennett MA, Carlson CE, et al: *Treatment of Pressure Ulcers. Clinical Practice Guideline, No. 15*. Rockville, Md, US Department of Health and Human Services, Public Health Service, Agency for Health Care Policy and Research, AHCPR Publication No. 95-0652, December 1994.

PART VI

Basic Science

CHAPTER 16

Gene Therapy for Vascular Disease

Michael J. Mann, M.D.
Instructor of Cardiovascular Medicine, Harvard Medical School,
Associate Physician, Brigham and Women's Hospital, Boston,
Massachusetts

Michael S. Conte, M.D.
Assistant Professor of Surgery, Harvard Medical School, Attending
Surgeon, Department of Surgery and Section of Vascular Surgery,
Brigham and Women's Hospital, Boston, Massachusetts

T he burgeoning "field" of gene therapy is barely a decade old. While physical and chemical methods of inserting foreign genes into mammalian cells have existed for some 25 years, the technical limitations of these approaches constrained them to laboratory investigation. The development of recombinant viral-based vector systems, beginning with the retrovirus in the 1980s, heralded the potential for therapeutic interventions. These systems, based on manipulation of the genome of a murine leukemia virus (Moloney; MMLV), allowed for the generation of recombinant, replication-defective particles capable of inserting genetic information in a safe and efficient manner.[1] The first approved clinical trial involving transfer of a foreign gene into humans, reported in 1990, used a retroviral vector to introduce a genetic marker to tumor-infiltrating lymphocytes ex vivo, as part of an immunotherapy protocol for advanced melanoma.[2]

Endothelial cells (ECs), by virtue of their location at the blood-tissue interface, were considered an attractive target for gene therapy from the outset. Methods for the reliable isolation and culture of human venous-derived ECs were developed in the 1970s, setting the stage for Herring and co-workers (1978) who first described a technique for implanting ("seeding") ECs on the surface of a prosthetic vascular graft in the hope of inducing a thromboresistant lining.[3] A decade later, although the original goal of this work remained in doubt, further investigations of EC seeding had greatly expanded the knowledge of interactions between ECs and biomaterials in vitro and in vivo. Reports of successful transduction of ECs with retroviral vectors[4] were followed shortly thereafter (1989) by the demonstration of successful implantation of genetically modified ECs in vivo on prosthetic vascular grafts[5] and balloon-injured arterial surfaces.[6] Limitations of retroviral vectors for direct in vivo gene delivery to the blood vessel wall, the most important of which is the requirement for target cell replication (see below), soon became readily apparent. This limitation is particularly relevant in the cardiovascular system, where the target cells (ECs, smooth muscle cells [SMCs]) normally have an exceedingly low rate of turnover. Early attempts to use retroviral vectors for direct transfer to arteries provided proof of concept but yielded rates of transduction that were too low for practical therapy.[7]

The advent of adenoviral vectors in the early 1990s provided a possible solution for in vivo gene delivery. Recombinant, replication-defective adenoviruses are highly stable particles that can be purified, concentrated to high titer, and are capable of efficiently infecting nondividing cells. Early studies in the cardiovascular system demonstrated relatively efficient transfer to endothelial cells in the intact vessel wall and to the heart.[8] Two major limiting factors subsequently emerged: limited duration of gene expression and host immunity. Adenoviruses do not integrate into the host cell's chromosomal DNA in their life cycle, a fact that may provide a safety advantage but that also prevents sustained gene expression when desired. More problematic is the significant host response to these viruses, which appears to consist of both nonspecific inflammation as well as direct antivector immunity. Significant local inflammation was observed after adenoviral exposure to blood vessels, inducing the expression of proadhesive molecules as well as a hyperplastic response in the arterial wall.[9] Minimizing the host response has become the major current focus of adenoviral vector development, with some progress being made by further deletion of nonessential, native viral genes. Newer generation adenoviral systems may be considerably less immunogenic, and are likely to be useful when brief but high- level gene expression is sufficient for the desired therapeutic effect.

The 1990s have also seen progressive development of other viral vector systems for gene therapy, including adeno-associated virus (AAV), herpesvirus, vaccinia, and lentivirus (HIV). Interest in AAV and lentiviral systems is primarily based on their ability to infect and integrate into nondividing cells, a critical parameter for most in vivo applications. Efforts to develop safe and efficient packaging systems are still in their earliest stages, particularly for lentivirus. A major recent impetus has been the concept of developing "hybrid" viruses, potentially incorporating desirable features of different viral types into new recombinant delivery particles. One example of this approach is the construction of "pseudotyped" retroviral vectors incorporating envelope proteins from other viruses (e.g., vesicular stomatitis virus [VSV]) that improve particle stability and amplify the range of target cell infectivity.[10]

Nonviral methods of gene delivery have also been a focus of intense development and progress during the last 5–10 years. Naked plasmid DNA, or plasmid-liposome complexes, are capable of transferring genetic sequences, albeit at extremely low efficiency (high number of particles required per target cell). Conversely they offer the potential advantages of excluding exogenous (i.e., viral) genetic information, relaxing gene size constraints, technical simplicity, and decreased host immune response. Mechanical force (e.g., pressure) may be required for efficient DNA transfer, although the mechanisms remain unclear. In some cell types (e.g., skeletal muscle), long-term expression has been documented with nonviral transfer.

Technological advances in catheters, stents, and local delivery systems have greatly enhanced the potential for direct applications of gene therapy in patients with cardiovascular disease. Access to the cardiovascular system, be it percutaneous or surgical, has become increasingly safe, sophisticated, and common in clinical practice. Although generally systemic in nature, most morbid complications of vascular diseases (e.g., atherosclerotic plaque rupture, restenosis after angioplasty, vein graft stenosis) occur at discrete, focal sites amenable to local therapies. In addition to considerations of access, the kinetic constraints of vector delivery to the vessel wall have led to the development of novel approaches, including hydrogel- coated balloon catheters, perforated catheters, double-balloon catheters, and periadventitial delivery systems.

Coupled with these technical advances in gene transfer and local delivery, a rapidly expanding knowledge of the molecular basis of vascular diseases has set the stage for genetic intervention. The last decade has seen the widespread use of genetic approaches in animal models of atherosclerosis, intimal hyperplasia, vein grafting, and angiogenesis. These investigations have broadly advanced the field of vascular biology by defining the role of specific genes in normal cardiovascular function as well as disease. In some cases, they have directly pointed the way to clinical gene therapy trials.

It seems clear that, as the new millenium approaches, improved delivery systems and an expanding array of molecular targets will lead to a growing role for genetic approaches in patients with cardiovascular disease.

BASIC CONCEPTS

PRINCIPLES OF GENE THERAPY

The advent of practical tools for carrying out gene therapy and genetic engineering strategies has created an avenue for the manipulation of disease at the level of its genetic blueprint. As molecular biologists have gained an increased understanding of the genetic switches that govern the onset and progression of specific diseases, clinical scientists have begun to consider ways of manipulating such processes to prevent, halt, or even reverse pathobiology at its roots, in a manner both more specific and more powerful than traditional pharmacotherapies. Genetic disorders linked to defective or missing gene products offer an obvious target for such intervention. The study of common, acquired diseases, however, has also revealed patterns of altered genetic activity in otherwise normal cells and tissues that may provide similarly effective targets for genetic manipulation. Such targets can include genes that encode proteins necessary for a disease process to become established; other targets may represent genes that support normal cellular biology and that are counteracted or suppressed during pathogenesis. Gene-based therapies can therefore include a spectrum of approaches including gene replacement, gene augmentation, new gene introduction, or gene blockade (Fig 1).

A cell's genetic material orchestrates its overall biological function, and each gene represents the code for the amino acid sequence of a particular protein. Gene expression refers to a process that begins with "transcription" of messenger RNA (mRNA) from the chromosomal DNA template, and leads to the "translation" of protein from the mRNA code. Transcription takes place in the mammalian cell nucleus, after which mRNA is transported to ribosomes located outside the nucleus for translation of protein. All cells within an individual carry an identical (or near identical) set of genes within their chromosomes; it is the pattern of expression of these genes in a differential manner that determines the morphology and biochemical function of different cells in different tissues. Just as this pattern of gene expression varies dramatically between "normal" cell types, thereby allowing a vascular SMC to look and act differently from a lymphocyte, neuron, or gastric parietal cell, changes

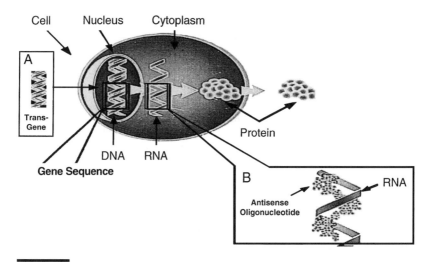

FIGURE 1.
Gene therapy strategies. Gene transfer involves delivery of an entire gene **(A)**, either by viral infection or by nonviral vectors, to the nucleus of a target cell. Expression of the gene via transcription into mRNA and translation into a protein gene product yields a functional protein that either achieves a therapeutic effect within the tranduced cell or is secreted to act on other cells. Gene blockade involves the introduction into the cell of short sequences of nucleic acids that block gene expression, such as antisense oligonucleotides **(B)** that bind mRNA in a sequence-specific fashion and prevent translation into protein.

in gene expression are being increasingly recognized as a fundamental event in triggering changes in cell behavior in diseased vs. healthy tissue.

GENE THERAPY STRATEGIES

Gene transfer involves the delivery of an intact gene into a living somatic cell. This genetic "construct" must contain regulatory elements (e.g., promoters and enhancers) that will enable expression of the gene once it has reached the cell nucleus. The transfer of a gene into a target cell leading to subsequent gene expression is known as *transduction*, and the new gene is often referred to as the *transgene*. "Transgenic" research differs from gene transfer in that transgenic animals have undergone insertion of a gene into the germ cell line, generally during embryogenesis of founder animals, so that this gene can be found in every cell of the transgenic organism. Although work with transgenic animals may provide a basis for development of clinical gene therapy strategies, actual human treatments will almost certainly require the transfer of genes into a subset of somatic cells in the patient after development.

The efficiency with which therapeutic gene transfer must be accomplished depends on the nature of the target gene. Gene *replacement* or *augmentation* involves the transfer of a gene that is either missing from a cell, present in a defective form, or simply underexpressed relative to the level of protein expression desired by the clinician. The protein expressed may be active only intracellularly, in which case a very high gene transfer efficiency must be achieved to alter the overall function of an organ or tissue. Alternatively, proteins secreted by target cells may act on other cells in a paracrine or endocrine manner, in which case delivery to a small subpopulation may yield a sufficient therapeutic result.

Gene *blockade* is another form of gene therapy that attempts to alter cellular function by the inhibition of specific gene expression. This may be accomplished using a variety of approaches. The most well-studied mechanism is the delivery of short chains of DNA known as antisense oligodeoxynucleotides (ODNs).[11] Genes are defined by the specific sequence of four bases, adenosine, thymidine, guanine, and cytosine, that make up the DNA chain. In the DNA double helix, adenosine subunits on one chain bind to thymidine subunits on the opposite chain, and the same is true of cytosine and guanine. This interaction of nucleic acid chains is known as "Watson-Crick" binding, and can occur between DNA and RNA chains as well. Antisense ODNs are designed to have a base sequence that is complementary in terms of Watson-Crick binding to a segment of the target gene. This complementary sequence allows the ODN to bind specifically to the corresponding segment of mRNA that is transcribed from the gene, preventing the translation of mRNA into the protein gene product.

Another form of gene blockade involves the use of "ribozymes," segments of RNA that can act like enzymes to destroy specific sequences of target mRNA.[12] Ribozymes contain both a catalytic region that can cleave other RNA molecules in a sequence-specific manner, and an adjacent sequence that confers the specificity of the target. A variety of ribozymes have been described that differ primarily in their three-dimensional structures. Because the sequence recognition portion of ribozymes is generally limited to approximately six bases, these gene inhibitory agents are generally more susceptible to nonspecific interactions than their antisense counterparts.

A third type of gene inhibition involves the blockade of gene regulatory proteins known as transcription factors. Transcription factors regulate gene expression by binding to chromosomal DNA at specific promoter regions, and this binding turns on, or "activates," an adjacent gene. Double-stranded ODNs can therefore be designed to mimic the chromosomal binding sites of these transcription factors and act as "decoys," binding up the available transcription factor and preventing the subsequent activation of target genes.[13]

In addition to gene replacement, augmentaton, and blockade, clinical strategies have been envisioned involving the transfer of genetic sequences exogenous to the human genome. An example is the gene encoding thymidine kinase (TK) from the herpes simplex virus, which has been used to enhance metabolic activation of the prodrug gancyclovir, inducing the death of TK-expressing cells. This approach of targeting cells for chemotherapy may be useful in neoplastic or vascular proliferative disorders (e.g., restenosis). Scientists studying gene transfer technology have often relied on a class of genes known as *reporter* or *marker genes*. These genes encode proteins, such as a form of β-galactosidase found in *Escherichia coli* (known as LacZ or β-gal), that can be detected easily via histochemical or other staining techniques and allow rapid identification and quantification of successful gene transfer.

Gene therapy can be carried out either in vivo in intact tissues, or in vitro in cell or organ culture. The former strategy depends on the safe delivery of transfection medium to the target cells within the patient. The latter approach, of course, requires the harvest of autologous or donor tissues or cells, a subsequent period of culture and transfection, and finally the effective reintroduction of the transfected material into the patient. While most vascular applications of gene therapy are likely to involve DNA delivery in vivo, strategies are also being explored for the reintroduction into target vessels of either endothelial or vascular SMCs that have been genetically modified in vitro.[14]

VECTORS

Although cells will take up DNA from their extracellular environment in small amounts, this uptake is inefficient and generally unsuitable to achieve a physiologically significant influence on the genetic function of either healthy or diseased tissue. Clinical gene therapies therefore depend on the development of vectors that enhance the efficiency of gene transfer both in vitro and in vivo. The "ideal" DNA delivery vector would be capable of safe and highly efficient delivery to all cell types, both proliferating and quiescent, with the opportunity to select either short-term or indefinite gene expression. This ideal vector would also have the flexibilty to accomodate genes of all sizes, incorporate control of the temporal pattern and degree of gene expression, and to recognize specific cell types for tailored delivery or expression. While progress is being made on each of these fronts individually, researchers remain far from possessing a single vector with all of these characteristics. Instead, a spectrum of vectors has evolved, each of which may find a niche in different early clinical gene therapy strategies. Following is a brief description of DNA delivery vectors that have been exploited in the vasculature (Table 1).

As in many contexts in medical science, nature has evolved systems for achieving the potential clinical goal of efficient gene transfer. Viruses are the most common vehicles for exogenous gene delivery into mammalian cells. Although they take on many distinct forms, all viruses consist of a genetic nucleic acid code encapsulated in a machinery that facilitates gene transfer and, in many cases, gene expression. Of course, every virus has developed a unique pattern of infection with regard to cell-type susceptibility and the size and makeup of the genetic material delivered. Recombinant DNA technology has allowed scientists to alter the genetic material contained within viral particles, both to include target genes of interest and to remove viral genes that contribute to host tissue toxicity.

Recombinant viral particles used as gene transfer vectors are distinguished from their naturally occurring derivative viruses by their inability to replicate (Fig 2). This is accomplished by deleting structural genes from the native viral genome that, in the normal virus life cycle, provide the blueprint for new virus production in infected host cells. Instead, these endogenous viral genes are replaced by the gene chosen for transfer, coupled to necessary regulatory elements using recombinant technology. To "package" these vectors into particles, cell lines are engineered to provide the missing structural viral proteins separately. The final vector particle is assembled to include the transgene construct as the only genetic information, with an otherwise normal external viral structure. These particles are therefore capable of efficient infection of suitable target cells when exposed, but cannot complete the intracellular life cycle of viral replication, exit from the cell, and further rounds of infection. Because the pathogenic effects of viruses are primarily related to these latter portions of the life cycle, direct toxicity to cells and tissues is generally minimal.

Although viral vectors represent nature's solution to the problem of efficient gene transfer, man's attempt to harness these

TABLE 1.

Comparison of Vector Types for Application to Cardiovascular Disease

	Efficiency (in vivo)	DNA Integration	Target Cells	Gene Size (max)	Particle Stability	Ease of Preparation	Host Response	Overall Applicability for CV Gene Therapy
Viral								
Retrovirus	+	+++++	Proliferating	8 kb	++++*	+++	+	++
Adenovirus	++++	0	Broad	8 kb†	++++	++	++++	+++
AAV	++	++++	Unknown	4 kb	++++	+	Unknown	Unknown
Nonviral								
Plasmid	+	+	Broad	≈50 kb	+++++	+++++	++‡	+
Plasmid-Lipid	+	+	Broad	≈50 kb	++	+++	+	+
Fusigenic Liposome	++ (variable)	+	Broad	≈50 kb	+	+	+	++

Note: +, lowest; +++++, highest.

N.B. Duration of expression in vivo is a complex issue that may vary for a given vector type depending on the transgene, method of delivery, tissue targeted, and species. In general, the intrinsic parameters of DNA integration and minimal host response are most clearly linked to prolonged expression.

*Pseudotyped retroviral particles incorporating vesicular stomatitis virus G-protein can be centrifuged to high titer without damage.

†Newer generations of "gutless" adenoviral vectors may fit in excess of 30 kB, but are difficult to prepare.

‡Some plasmid preparations may be highly immunogenic. Variability in host response is likely to be transgene specific.

Abbreviations: CV, cardiovascular; *AAV,* adeno-associated virus.

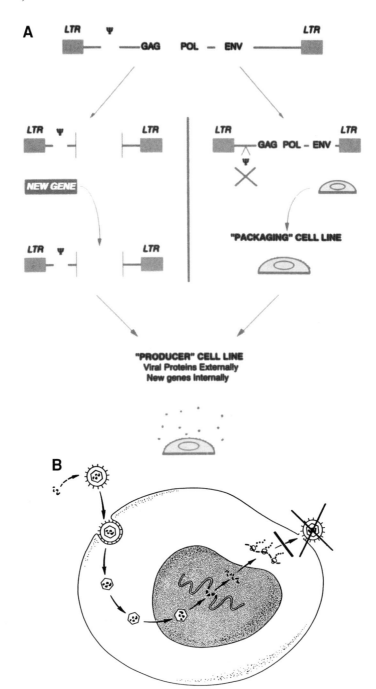

resources has also been confounded by the biological barriers that have evolved to protect cells and organisms from viral infection. Immunologic responses not only limit the efficacy of viral gene transfer, particularly when repeat administrations are considered, but the inflammatory response to viral antigens, even those associated with replication-deficient vectors, may impede or negate the benefits of expression of the transfered gene. Furthermore, engineering of viral genomes does not always preclude residual cytotoxicty in infected cells, and the possibility for regression to replication proficiency or for further mutation and recombination with other virulent viruses in the environment pose biological hazards that are difficult to quantitate or predict.

Scientists have therefore continued to explore nonviral avenues for achieving efficient DNA delivery. One advantage of nonviral delivery systems is that they can be used not only for gene transfer, but also for delivery of oligonucleotides and protein–nucleic acid complexes that can be used for alternative forms of genetic manipulation. Whereas *transduction* refers generally to the delivery of an intact gene to a target cell, and infection is used to describe the process of viral gene delivery, *transfection* is a term used to describe nonviral (i.e., physical/chemical) delivery of genes or oligonucleotides.

Retroviral Vectors

Retroviruses contain RNA genomes, and express an enzyme, known as reverse transcriptase, that generates double-stranded

---

FIGURE 2.
Generation of recombinant retroviral particles for gene transfer. **A,** the MMLV genome is depicted schematically. There are 3 major viral gene products encoded by the genes *gag, pol,* and *env.* At either end of the single-stranded RNA genome are long-terminal repeat *(LTR)* sequences that contain important regulatory elements. The ψ-sequence is a packaging signal that must be present for encapsidation of viral constructs. Gene transfer constructs *(left-hand side)* are made by removing the structural genes and inserting the gene of interest downstream from ψ. These constructs are then transfected into a stable "packaging cell" line made by transfection of the ψ-deleted genomic elements. A "producer cell" line is thus created that yields recombinant viral particles devoid of the structural genetic information, and containing the transgene. **B,** interaction of a retroviral vector with a target cell demonstrates receptor-mediated binding, uncoating, reverse transcription, and integration of the virally introduced gene into the chromosome. Transcription and translation now produce only the desired protein gene product; no new virus can be formed. (Courtesy of Louis K. Birinyi, M.D.)

DNA from the viral RNA template. This DNA is then inserted into the chromosomal genome of the host cell, from which it is expressed. For this insertion to take place, the infected cell must undergo cell division within a short time after infection, so that traditional retroviruses can deliver DNA effectively only to actively replicating cells. Once viral gene insertion has taken place, this exogenous genetic material continues to be passed on to subsequent generations of progeny cells, creating the possibility for stable gene expression. Recombinant, replication-deficient retroviral vectors have been used extensively for gene transfer in cultured cells in vitro, where cell proliferation can be easily manipulated. Their use in vivo has been more limited because of low transduction efficiencies, particularly in the vascular system where most cells remain quiescent. Nabel et al.[7] first demonstrated the feasibility of transducing blood vessels with foreign DNA in vivo by infecting porcine iliofemoral arteries with a recombinant retroviral vector containing the β-galactosidase gene. Several cell types in the vessel wall were transduced, including endothelial and vascular SMCs. Using a β-galactosidase retroviral vector to genetically modify endothelial cells in vitro, Wilson et al.[5] demonstrated β-galactosidase expression up to 5 weeks after implantation of prosthetic vascular grafts seeded with genetically transformed cells. The random integration of traditional retroviral vectors such as MMLV into chromosomal DNA represents a potential hazard that could lead to dysregulated cell growth. While the risk appears to be exceedingly low, this remains an important area for safety monitoring in clinical trials.

Recent improvements in packaging systems (particularly the development of "pseudotyped" retroviral vectors incorporating the VSV G-protein) have improved the stability of retroviral particles and facilitated their use. Recombinant retroviral supernatant can now be generated in large batches, concentrated to high titer, and stored frozen until use, without significant loss of infectivity. No additional special preparation is required at the time of use, other than to thaw and mix the virus with polybrene or a similar adjuvant.

Adenoviral Vectors

Recombinant adenoviruses have become the most widely used viral vectors for in vivo gene transfer, and have been used extensively in experimental cardiovascular systems.[15] Adenoviruses can infect nondividing cells and generally do not integrate into the host genome. These vectors can therefore achieve relatively efficient gene transfer in quiescent vascular tissue, but transgenes are generally lost when cells are stimulated into rounds of cell division. Expression of DNA in a nonchromosomal, or episomal, state also appears to be less stable, and adenoviral transduction has proven to be transient in cells even in the absence of replication. A number of different adenoviral serotypes exist, and although most recombinant gene transfer vectors are based on serotype 5, it has been proposed that different serotypes could be used to allow repeat administrations to avoid neutralization by the host immune response. Most experimental adenoviral vectors have undergone deletion of the viral genes known as E1a and E1b—genes that play an early critical role in the adenoviral replication cycle—to render the vectors replication-deficient. The E3 region has also been deleted, providing enough space in the recombinant genome for inserting DNA of up to 7.5 kb. Researchers are currently exploring removal of nearly all adenoviral genes both to reduce the immunogenicity of the vector and to increase the size of possible transgene insertions.

Many scientists have concluded that the immune response to adenoviral antigens represents the greatest limitation to their use in gene therapy. Conventional vectors have generally achieved gene expression for only 1–2 weeks after infection. It is not certain to what degree the destruction of infected cells contributes to the termination of transgene expression, and suppression of activity of episomal transgene promoters also appears to play a role. However, longer expression has been documented after infection of tissues in immune deficient mice. The role of immune reactions against the transgene protein product itself has also attracted increasing attention, as researchers are recognizing the need for species compatibility of the therapeutic protein. Even in the context of such reactions, the adenoviral vector has been postulated to provide an adjuvant effect that amplifies the immune response. In the vasculature, physical barriers have also been found to limit the effectiveness of adenoviral gene transfer. In intact vessels, the internal elastic lamina apparently limits infection to the endothelium, with gene transfer to the media and adventitia only occuring after injury has disrupted the vessel architecture. Although gene delivery to 30% to 60% of cells after balloon injury has been reported with adenoviral vectors carrying reporter genes, the fact that atherosclerotic disease has also been found to limit the efficiency of adenoviral transduction may pose a significant problem for the treatment of human disease.

Another practical limitation to the use of adenoviral vectors as experimental tools is the complexity and time-consuming nature of adenoviral vector construction. An alternative method of using adenoviral gene transfer is also under investigation: coupling of adenoviral particles to transferrin-polylysine/DNA complexes. Using the endosome-disruptive activity of inactivated adenovirus particles and poly-L-lysine, gene constructs (up to 48 kb) have been transfected with high efficiency in vitro and in vivo to autologous rabbit jugular vein grafts.[16] Complexing unmodified plasmid DNA with replication-deficient adenovirus via cationic lipids has been reported to enhance gene transfer both in vitro and in vivo.

Adenoviral vectors are produced in batches, concentrated to high titer, and stored frozen until use. Infective titer is well maintained and reproducible. No special handling procedures are required at the time of application, making them potentially simple to use in clinical settings.

Adeno-Associated Viral Vectors

Adeno-associated virus is a dependent human parvovirus that is not able to replicate unless a helper virus, such as adenovirus or herpes virus, is present in the same cell.[17] Adeno-associated virus has not been linked to human disease. It can infect a wide range of target cell lines, and can establish a latent infection by integration into the genome of the cell, thereby yielding stable gene transfer as in the case of retroviral vectors. Although AAV vectors transduce replicating cells at a more rapid rate, they possess the ability to infect nonreplicating cells both in vitro and in vivo. Adeno-associated virus is limited by its small size (transgenes cannot be longer than about 4 kb), and the need to eliminate helper viruses from viral preparations. Early applications of AAV vectors to human gene therapy have included phenotypic correction of Fanconi anemia in human hematopoietic cells, and stable in vivo expression of the cystic fibrosis transmembrane conductance regulator in airway epithelial cells. The efficiency of AAV-mediated gene transfer to vascular cells, and the potential use of AAV vectors for in vivo vascular gene therapy remain to be determined.

Lipid-Mediated Gene Transfer

Numerous nonviral methods are available for the delivery of DNA into cells in vitro, including calcium phosphate, electroporation, and particle bombardment. The development of similarly effective methods of in vivo transfection, however, has posed a significant challenge to cardiovascular and other clinical researchers who hope to avoid cumbersome and invasive steps of harvesting and culturing tissues or cells from the patient. The encapsulation of DNA in artificial lipid membranes (liposomes) can facilitate its uptake and cellular transport. The primary advantages of lipid-based gene transfer methods are ease of preparation and flexibility in substituting different transgene constructs in comparison with the relatively complex process of producing recombinant viral vectors. Cationic liposomes have been used extensively during the last 5 years for cellular delivery of plasmid DNA and antisense oligonucleotides.[18] The activity of cationic liposomes is thought to be mediated by (1) spontaneous capture of the negatively charged polynucleotides with cationic lipids by a condensation reaction; (2) increased cellular uptake resulting from interaction of positively charged complexes with negatively charged biological membranes; and (3) membrane fusion (or transient membrane destabilization) with the plasmalemma or the endosome to achieve delivery into the cytoplasm while avoiding degradation in the lysosomal compartment. Recent data indicate that movement of DNA from the cytoplasm to the nucleus and successful dissociation of DNA from the lipid complex appear to be important variables for lipid-mediated gene transfer, and expression of recombinant genes after cationic lipid-mediated gene transfer has been demonstrated in vivo in several animal models.

A wide variety of cationic lipid preparations are currently available for DNA transfer both in vitro and in vivo. Each is composed of a mixture of neutral and cationic lipid, and each differs slightly in its spectrum of activity in terms of susceptible cell types, resistance to serum exposure, and stability. Although widespread transgene expression has been reported after intravenous injection of some cationic lipid-plasmid DNA formulations, consistently efficient transfection in vivo with cationic lipids has yet to be established. Early clinical trials with cationic lipid:DNA complexes have focused primarily on direct injection into malignant tumors, such as metastatic melanoma, to induce a heightened antitumor immunologic response. In addition to cationic lipids, other substances such as lipopolyamines and cationic polypeptides are now being investigated as potential vehicles for enhanced DNA delivery both for gene transfer and gene blockade strategies.

Recently, researchers have explored enhancing the properties of nonviral gene transfer vectors. Efficiency of gene delivery has been found to correlate with the supercoiling of DNA and its trafficking within the cell. Complexing of DNA with various histone and other nonhistone nuclear proteins has been found to assist DNA compaction and improve nuclear localization. Cell targeting and increased delivery is also being developed through the insertion of cell-specific antibodies and cell-specific receptor ligands into lipid:DNA complexes. The concept of an "artificial virus" involves packaging a collection of genes encoding enzymes, such as RNA polymerases, and other proteins that can mediate transgene expression as well as amplify their own expression. Such a packaging system might facilitate cytopolasmic expression of transgenes and reduce dependence on endogenous cellular gene expression machinery and its complex regulation. In addition, self-replicating plasmids, into which viral sequences have been cloned that trigger initiation of DNA synthesis, may allow long-term transgene expression that is similar to what has been achieved after retroviral vector infection.

Fusigenic–Liposome-Mediated Gene Transfer (HVJ-Liposomes)

This method uses a combination of fusigenic proteins of the Sendai virus (hemagglutinating virus of Japan [HVJ]) in conjunction with neutral liposomes. Hemagglutinating virus of Japan is an RNA virus and belongs to the paramyxovirus family, which has HN and F glycoproteins on its envelope.[19] The HN glycoprotein binds with glycol-type sialic acid groups that act as receptors on the cell surface, and F protein can interact directly with the cellular lipid bilayer and induce fusion. HVJ-liposomes consist of neutral liposomes complexed with ultraviolet light–inactivated HVJ virus. Fusion of HVJ liposome complexes with the cell membrane may result in the release of DNA directly into the cytosol, bypassing endocytosis, thereby reducing lysosomal destruction of the DNA construct and facilitating nuclear uptake. HVJ-liposome methods have been successfully used for gene transfer in vivo to many tissues including liver, kidney, and the vascular wall. A major limitation to current HVJ-liposome techniques is the need to undertake a multistep liposome preparation procedure immediately before use because of the poor long-term stability of the complexes.

Other In Vivo Gene Transfer Methods

Plasmids are circular chains of DNA that were originally discovered as a natural means of gene transfer between bacteria. Naked plasmids can also be used to transfer DNA into mammalian cells. The direct injection of plasmid DNA into tissues in vivo can result in transgene expression. Plasmid uptake and expression, however, has generally been achieved at reasonable levels only in skeletal and myocardial muscle.[20] The uptake of naked oligonucleotides is also inefficient after either intravascular administration or direct injection. Various catheters that have been designed to enhance local drug delivery to isolated segments of target vessels have been proposed as vehicles for local gene therapy. The controlled application of a pressurized environment to vascular tissue in a nondistending manner has recently been found to enhance oligonucleotide uptake and nuclear localization. This method may be particularly useful for ex vivo applications such as vein grafting or transplantation, and may represent a means of enhancing plasmid gene delivery as well.[21]

SPECIFIC APPROACHES IN VASCULAR DISEASE

Many vascular diseases represent systemic disorders, and metabolic and physiologic factors are now known to contribute to their onset and progression. Although the significance of genetic factors for elements of vascular pathogenesis, such as hyperlipidemia and hypertension, is slowly emerging, a role for gene-based therapies in modifying these factors remains primarily speculative at present. A model for future interventions, however, may be the experimental and early clinical experience in treating the genetic form of familial hypercholesterolemia caused by a defect in the low-density lipoprotein (LDL) receptor. This receptor facilitates LDL uptake in the liver and is essential for maintaining normal cholesterol levels. Genetic replacement of this missing protein in liver cells has been accomplished in a rabbit model of LDL receptor deficiency via surgical harvest of autologous liver cells, stable transduction in vitro with a retroviral vector, and reinfusion of the cells via the portal circulation. These results formed the basis of a subsequent clinical trial of this method of gene therapy in human subjects. More recently, adenoviral vectors have been used for in vivo gene transfer of lipoprotein receptor genes into similar animal models of hypercholesterolemia without the need for the invasive harvest and culture of autologus cells. Vascular gene therapy, however, is more likely to find early widespread application in the treatment or prevention of focal lesions.

GENETIC ENGINEERING OF FAILURE-RESISTANT VEIN GRAFTS

The long-term success of surgical revascularization in the lower extremity and coronary circulations has been limited by significant rates of autologous vein graft failure. No pharmacologic approach has been successful at preventing long- term graft diseases such as neointimal hyperplasia or graft atherosclerosis. Gene therapy offers a new avenue for the modification of vein graft biology that might lead to a reduction in clinical morbidity from graft failures. Intraoperative transfection of the vein graft also offers an opportunity to combine intact tissue DNA transfer techniques with the increased safety of ex vivo transfection, and a number of studies have documented the feasibility of ex vivo gene transfer into vein grafts using viral vectors.

The vast majority of vein graft failures have been linked to the neointimal disease that is part of graft remodeling after surgery. Although neointimal hyperplasia contributes to the reduction of wall stress in vein grafts after bypass, this process can also lead to luminal narrowing of the graft conduit during the first years after operation. Furthermore, the abnormal neointimal layer, with its production of proinflammatory proteins, is believed to form the basis for an accelerated form of graft atherosclerosis that causes late graft failure. An ex vivo ODN transfection approach has been designed that would inhibit neointimal hyperplasia and thereby yield resistance to graft disease and failure.[22]

In preclinical studies, rabbit vein grafts were transfected at the time of surgery with ODNs that blocked SMC proliferation and neointimal hyperplasia after grafting. This blockade was achieved via inhibition of gene expression necessary for progression of VSMC through the cell cycle toward cell division. Initially, it was found that a combination of antisense ODNs that inhibit expression of at least two cell-cycle regulatory genes could significantly block neointimal hyperplasia. An alternative approach in which a decoy ODN was designed to block the activity of a critical transcription factor (known as E2F), subsequently yielded similar efficacy with a single, more potent agent. E2F is responsible for the coordinated expression of up to a dozen genes during the critical early stages of progression through cell-cycle check points. In contrast to arterial balloon injury, however, vein grafts are not only subjected to a single injury at the time of operation, but are also exposed to chronic hemodynamic stimuli for remodeling. Despite these chronic stimuli, a single, intraoperative ODN treatment of vein grafts resulted in a resistance to neointimal hyperplasia that lasted for at least 6 months in the rabbit model. During that period, the grafts treated with antisense ODNs were able to adapt to arterial conditions via hypertrophy of the medial layer. Furthermore, these genetically engineered conduits proved resistant to diet-induced graft atherosclerosis (Fig 3) and were associated with preserved endothelial function.

A large-scale, prospective, randomized, double-blind trial of human vein graft treatment with E2F decoy ODNs has recently been initiated. Efficient delivery of ODNs is accomplished within 15 minutes during the operation by placement of the graft after harvest in a device that exposes the vessel to ODNs in physiologic solution and creates a nondistending pressurized environment of 300

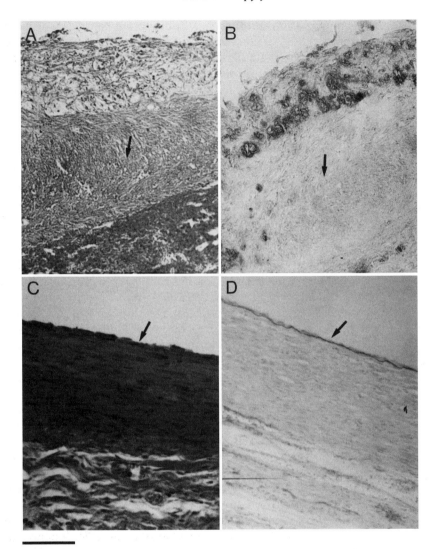

FIGURE 3.

Cell-cycle inhibition alters remodeling of experimental vein grafts in rabbits. Light micrographs of control oligodeoxynucleotide (ODN)-treated **(A and B)** and antisense ODN-treated **(C and D)** vein grafts in hypercholesterolemic rabbits 6 weeks after surgery. *Arrows* indicate the location of the internal elastic lamina. Macrophages are identified immunohistochemically **(B)** in a foam cell lesion corresponding to macroscopic plaque in a control graft. Neointimal hyperplasia is significantly inhibited in the antisense ODN-treated graft, which instead has undergone an adaptive process of medial hypertrophy and has remained free of plaque or macrophage invasion.

mm Hg (Fig 4, A). Preliminary findings indicate ODN delivery to greater then 80% of graft cells, and effective blockade of target gene expression (Fig 4, B). This study will measure the effect of cell-cycle gene blockade on primary graft failure rates, and represents one of the first attempts to definitively determine the feasibility of clinical genetic manipulation in the treatment of a common cardiovascular disorder.

POSTANGIOPLASTY RESTENOSIS

Recurrent narrowing of arteries after percutaneous angioplasty, atherectomy, or other disobliterative techniques is a common clinical problem that severely limits the durability of these procedures for patients with atherosclerotic occlusive diseases. In the case of balloon angioplasty, restenosis occurs in approximately 30% to 40% of treated coronary lesions and 30% to 50% of superficial femoral artery lesions within the first year. Intravascular stents may reduce the restenosis rate in some settings; however, the incidence remains significant and long-term data are limited. Despite impressive technological advances in the development of minimally invasive and endovascular approaches to treat arterial occlusions, the full benefit of these gains awaits the resolution of this fundamental biological problem.

Restenosis is an attractive target for gene therapy not only because of its frequency (and the associated costs incurred on the health care system), but more so because it is a local tissue reaction that develops precisely at a site of intervention to which access has been accomplished. An assumed advantage of the genetic approach over more conventional pharmacotherapies is that a single dose of agent may have a protracted biological effect. It has been reasoned that the appropriate genetic modification, performed locally at the time of angioplasty, could induce a long-term benefit in patency by altering the healing response. The potential role for gene therapy in the prevention of restenosis will depend on the identification of an appropriate molecular target, a suitable vector system for efficiently targeting vessel wall cells, and methods of achieving local delivery without producing undue damage or distal tissue ischemia. Presently, considerable hurdles remain despite significant progress in each of these areas.

The pathophysiology of restenosis reflects a paradigm of the healing response of arteries that are injured by reconstructive techniques. The pathologic hallmark of restenosis is intimal hyperplasia, a flow-restricting fibrocellular lesion composed primarily of SMCs and extracellular matrix. Experimental studies using animal

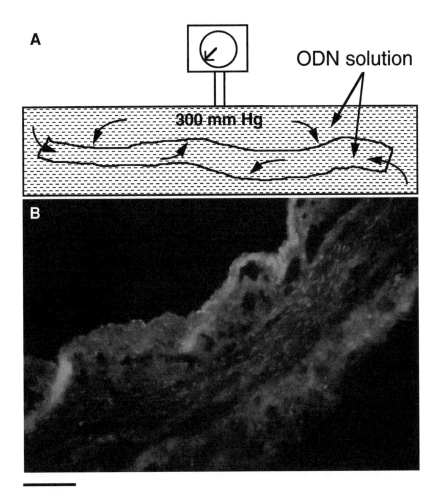

FIGURE 4.

Intraoperative transfection of vein bypass grafts. **A,** schematic of intraoperative delivery method. Grafts are mounted on a device that allows exposure to oligodeoxynucleotide *(ODN)* solution (both intraluminally and extraluminally) at 300 mm Hg in a *nondistending* manner. **B,** intra-operative, pressure-mediated delivery of fluorescent-labeled ODNs to vein graft cells. Cross-section of segment of saphenous vein 2 hours after exposure to labeled ODNs by above method (viewed under fluorescein isothiocyanate [FITC]-epifluorescence; original magnification, ×100). Note the pattern of enhanced green fluorescence in the nuclei of cells within the graft wall, indicating nuclear localization of labeled ODNs.

models of arterial injury have demonstrated a temporal sequence of SMC proliferation, migration, phenotypic change, and matrix production in the developing intimal lesion. Despite the significant knowledge gained from these studies of neointimal lesion formation, numerous recent clinical observations have called into question the importance of the neointima in postangioplasty restenosis. It now appears that constrictive remodeling, as opposed to neointimal mass, accounts for the majority of late lumen loss after balloon dilation of atherosclerotic vessels. The process of vascular remodeling has only recently become a focus of intense scientific investigation, and the critical cellular and molecular signals have yet to be elucidated. The development of more appropriate animal models will be critical in these efforts. Thus the question of choosing an appropriate molecular target, based on a clear understanding of the biological process of restenosis, must still be considered as the primary obstacle to developing a clinically effective genetic approach.

Despite these caveats, proliferation has been the predominant target of experimental genetic interventions. There have been two general approaches: "cytostatic," in which cells are prevented from progressing through the cell cycle to mitosis, and cytotoxic, where actual cell death is induced. Examples of the former include engineered overexpression of intrinsic cell-cycle inhibitors, dominant mutant forms of critical cell-cycle proteins (e.g., retinoblastoma protein) that block activity of the native normal protein, antisense oligonucleotides to block expression of critical cell-cycle regulatory genes, autocrine/paracrine inhibitors of SMC growth (e.g., nitric oxide), and transcription factor "decoys." An example of a direct cytotoxic approch is the transfer of a "suicide gene" such as the herpesvirus TK gene that has already been mentioned. All of these approaches have been used with success in animal models of injury-induced neointima formation, demonstrating a local antiproliferative effect of gene transfer.

Another potentially relevant biological target is reendothelialization, which might be accelerated by local delivery of a proangiogenic cytokine (e.g., vascular endothelial growth factor [VEGF]) at the angioplasty site. This is the basis for the only current U.S. clinical trial of gene therapy for the prevention of restenosis in the peripheral circulation, in which the human VEGF gene is administered as a "naked" circular DNA plasmid directly to the injured arterial wall on the surface of the angioplasty balloon.[23] The investigators hypothesize that the low efficiency of this delivery method is balanced by the high biological potency of this secreted angiogenic cytokine, enabling a significant local biological effect despite poor gene transfer.

Successful and efficient gene transfer to the injured, atherosclerotic arterial wall presents unique mechanical and kinetic challenges. For strategies designed to attenuate or prevent SMC proliferation, the target cell mass lies within the media of the vessel wall. After balloon angioplasty, mechanical disruption and dissection of plaque may facilitate particle delivery to deeper layers of the vessel wall; however, uniform delivery to the bulk of target SMCs is problematic and may require high intraluminal pressure or other mechanical forces. Experimental models of neointima formation in animals may not be clinically relevant given their high, uniform cellular content and absence of the more predominant noncellular components of complex atherosclerotic plaque in humans. Kinetic constraints on delivery are significant as well. Transfer of genetic material requires significant contact time between particles and target cells, mandating innovative approaches at the interface with flowing blood. In the coronary circulation, prolonged dwell times under vascular occlusion may not be practical without some mechanism for distal perfusion. This would clearly be less of an issue in peripheral arteries. Sustained release gels or matrices may provide other solutions to the delivery problem, either intraluminal or periadventitial.

The ex vivo approach, with implantation of genetically modified ECs or SMCs at sites of arterial injury, is also being investigated (Fig 5). The necessity for harvesting autologous donor tissue for target cells, coupled with the increased costs and complexity of tissue culture, have greatly dampened the enthusiasm for this strategy in favor of more direct methods. Nonetheless, it remains clinically feasible and, in the case of ECs, the implanted cells alone may confer beneficial properties to the healing arterial wall. Application of these cell transplantation approaches would be greatly facilitated by the development of "universal donor" cell lines in which major histocompatibility antigens have been "knocked out." Such a development, while clearly years or decades away, may no longer be merely science fiction fantasy.

In summary, it would appear that the application of gene therapy for postangioplasty restenosis may still be somewhat premature.[24] In addition to major obstacles in delivering genes to the atherosclerotic vessel wall (including both vector and catheter-device constraints), the fundamental biological process remains incompletely understood. Nonetheless, continued progress on each of these fronts warrants an optimistic view for genetic approaches

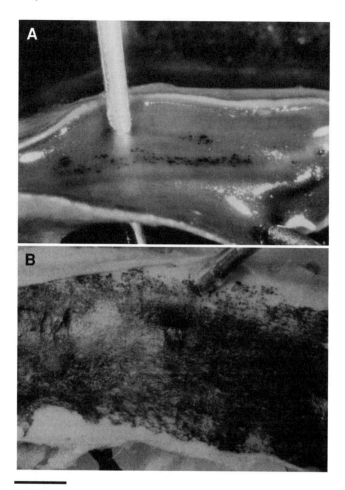

FIGURE 5.

Retroviral-mediated gene transfer to rabbit arterial endothelium. **A,** direct in vivo exposure of a rabbit iliac artery to recombinant retrovirus containing the β-galactosidase gene. The vessel was minimally injured using a fine-wire loop 2 days before virus exposure to stimulate endothelial proliferation. Expression of the transgene, indicated by the blue reaction product, is evident in a small number of endothelial cells (ECs) 1 week after infection. **B,** endothelial cell seeding approach. Venous ECs were harvested from rabbit jugular vein and exposed to the identical β-galactosidase vector particles in vitro. Two weeks later, the cells were implanted on the surface of an acutely injured (balloon catheter) iliac artery. En face view of artery stained for β-galactosidase activity 1 week later shows almost complete relining with genetically modified ECs. In this model, transgene expression is variable at 2 weeks and lost at 1 month.

to control the arterial injury response. These developments will undoubtedly yield important corollaries for the surgical treatment of arterial occlusive diseases as well.

THERAPEUTIC ANGIOGENESIS

A recent explosion in knowledge of the molecular signals involved in normal and pathologic blood vessel growth has fueled considerable interest in clinical applications of angiogenesis research. The potential of augmenting collateral blood vessel formation as a means of improving perfusion of ischemic extremities or end organs (e.g., myocardium) has long been debated and is now being investigated in the clinic. A number of groups have initiated preliminary, phase I studies involving delivery of proangiogenic molecules to ischemic myocardium, either as direct protein injections or by injection of genetic constructs encoding these proteins. A gene therapy clinical trial is currently underway in patients with end-stage lower extremity occlusive disease who are not candidates for traditional revascularization options.[25] In this protocol, the plasmid encoding the human VEGF gene is delivered by multiple injections into the calf musculature. Preliminary results suggest minimal toxicity. (Despite premature reports in the news media suggesting clear-cut evidence of benefit, this study is a phase I, uncontrolled trial that is designed primarily to assess safety.)

More clinical trials of angiogenic agents will likely follow, particularly in the coronary circulation. Significant questions of duration of effect, hemodynamic benefit, and potential for uncontrolled blood vessel growth (i.e., hemangioma formation) will be critical issues for careful study, which should primarily be carried out in experimental animal models. While numerous animal studies have suggested augmentation of collateral vessel formation in ischemic limbs/organs after delivery of angiogenic genes (e.g., VEGF), it is important to point out that the models used are largely those of acute, not chronic ischemia. As in the case of vasodilator therapy for chronic arterial occlusive disease, where the loss of autoregulation (e.g., the ruborous foot) indicates maximal intrinsic vasodilation and a low likelihood of response to further pharmacology, so it may be that chronically ischemic tissue is already maximally upregulated in local production of angiogenic cytokines. Further studies will be required to determine the pathophysiologic settings in which therapeutic angiogenesis may be clinically useful; however, it appears likely that this will be a productive area for gene transfer approaches in the decade ahead.

PROSTHETIC VASCULAR GRAFTS

Poor long-term patency severely limits the application of currently available synthetic grafts as small-caliber (6 mm) arterial substitutes. Gene therapy has been envisioned as a potential avenue for altering the host-biomaterial interactions in a favorable way. Seeding genetically modified ECs (or SMCs) to prosthetic graft surfaces may allow for therapeutic manipulation of local surface properties, inflammatory responses, and tissue ingrowth. Proteins having antithrombotic, thrombolytic, antiproliferative, and angiogenic properties are all potentially relevant targets for this type of approach. As in the other pathologic states discussed above, a major limiting factor is the state of our knowledge of the molecular events involved in prosthetic graft failure. Most such grafts occlude because of progressive perianastomotic thickening of the recipient vessel, leading to severe flow restriction; this process is still poorly understood. Nonetheless, addressing the final common pathways of thrombosis and inflammation might feasibly extend graft patency, even if the underlying process is only partially affected.

Experience with EC seeding of prosthetics has strongly suggested that the establishment of a durable, flow-resistant lining of cells on the surface of a prosthetic requires a period of in vitro culture on the biomaterial. This requirement, in addition to the need for adequate numbers of autologous donor cells, is the most significant technical obstacle limiting clinical application. Recent reports of successful isolation and expansion of endothelial precursors from peripheral blood may provide a solution to the issue of donor tissue. Continued refinements of biomaterials, precoating substrates, and techniques will be required to perform graft seeding in a single, intraoperative step without experiencing high rates of subsequent cell loss upon exposure to flow. These practical obstacles to cell seeding are the most critical, and new solutions will be required before additional genetic interventions are likely to make a clinical impact on prosthetic graft occlusion.

CONCLUSIONS

Gene therapy has become a clinical reality, if only in its most primordial forms at present. Its premise is based firmly on the knowledge of the genetic basis of normal and abnormal cellular function, a knowledge that grows at an astounding pace and will be amplified by the expected completion of the full sequencing of the human genome. The greatest challenge ahead for molecular medicine will be the assimilation and integration of this large volume of data, and the development of information systems capable of linking a multitude of patterns of gene expression with cellular phenotype and organ (dys)function. The complexity of most pathophysiologic processes at the molecular level may require multigene approaches to maintain normal tissue function. Nonetheless the die has been cast, and the future for interventions at the genetic level is bright.

Current limitations of gene therapy for cardiovascular disease are significant but surmountable. Improved vector systems, catheter technology, and biocompatible polymers are likely to solve many of the problems of delivery enumerated above. Genetic approaches will only be successful if based on a thorough understanding of the molecular basis of pathophysiologic states. Because of their ability to obtain uncomplicated access to the cardiovascular system, surgeons are likely to play a critically important, early role in the initial development of clinical applications. Vein graft disease, long the bane of the vascular surgeon, leads the list of pathologic entities ripe for genetic intervention. Vehicles for delivering genes to blood vessels may one day be as commonplace and indispensable in the operating room as heparin is today.

REFERENCES

1. Danos O, Mulligan RC: Safe and efficient generation of recombinant retroviruses with amphotropic and ecotropic host ranges. *Proc Natl Acad Sci USA* 85:6460–6464, 1988.
2. Rosenberg SA, Aebersold P, Cometta K, et al: Gene transfer into humans: Immunotherapy of patients with advanced melanoma using tumor-infiltrating lymphocytes modified by retroviral gene transduction. *N Engl J Med* 323:570–578, 1990.
3. Herring M, Gardner A, Glover J: A single staged technique for seeding vascular grafts with autogenous endothelium. *Surgery* 84:498–504, 1978.
4. Zweibel JA, Freeman SM, Kantoff PW, et al: High-level recombinant gene expression in rabbit endothelial cells transduced by retroviral vectors. *Science* 243:220–222, 1989.
5. Wilson JM, Birinyi LK, Salomon RN, et al: Implantation of vascular grafts lined with genetically modified endothelial cells. *Science* 244:1344–1346, 1989.
6. Nabel EG, Plautz G, Boyce FM, et al: Recombinant gene expression in-vivo within endothelial cells of the arterial wall. *Science* 244:1342–1343, 1989.
7. Nabel EG, Plautz G, Nabel GJ: Site-specific gene expression in-vivo by direct gene transfer into the arterial wall. *Science* 249:1285–1288, 1990.

8. Lemarchand P, Jones M, Yamada I, et al: In vivo gene transfer and expression in normal uninjured blood vessels using replication-deficient recombinant adenovirus vectors. *Circ Res* 72:1132–1138, 1993.

9. Newman KD, Dunn PF, Owens JW, et al: Adenovirus-mediated gene transfer into normal rabbit arteries results in prolonged vascular cell activation, inflammation, and neointimal hyperplasia. *J Clin Invest* 96:2955–2965, 1995.

10. Ory DS, Neugeboren BA, Mulligan RC. A stable human-derived packaging cell line for production of high titer retrovirus/vesicular stomatitis virus G pseudotypes. *Proc Natl Acad Sci USA* 93:11400–11406, 1996.

11. Colman A. Antisense strategies in cell and developmental biology. *J Cell Sci* 97:399–409, 1990.

12. Zaug A, Been M, Cech T: The Tetrahymena ribozyme acts like an RNA restriction endonuclease. *Nature* 324:429–433, 1986.

13. Bielinska A, Schivdasani RA, Zhang L, et al: Regulation of gene expression with double-stranded phosphothioate oligonucleotides. *Science* 250:997–1000, 1990.

14. Conte MS, Birinyi LK, Miyata T, et al: Efficient repopulation of denuded rabbit arteries with autologous genetically modified endothelial cells. *Circulation* 89:2161–2169, 1994.

15. Brody SL, Crystal RG: Adenovirus-mediated in vivo gene transfer. *Ann N Y Acad Sci* 716:90–101, 1994.

16. Kupfer JM, Ruan XM, Liu G, et al: High-efficiency gene transfer to autologous rabbit jugular vein grafts using adenovirus-transferrin/polylysine-DNA complexes. *Hum Gene Ther* 5:1437–1443, 1994.

17. Muzyczka N: Use of adeno-associated virus as a general transduction vector for mammalian cells. *Curr Top Microbiol Immunol* 158:97–129, 1992.

18. Felgner PL, Gader TR, Holm M, et al: Lipofectin: A highly efficient, lipid mediated DNA-transfection procedure. *Proc Natl Acad Sci USA* 84:7413–7417, 1987.

19. Dzau VJ, Mann MJ, Morishita R, et al: Fusigenic viral liposome for gene therapy in cardiovascular diseases. *Proc Natl Acad Sci USA* 93:11421–11425, 1996.

20. Lin H, Parmacek MS, Morle G, et al: Expression of recombinant gene in myocardium in vivo after direct injection of DNA. *Circulation* 82:2217–2221, 1990.

21. Mann MJ, Whittemore AD, Donaldson MC, et al: Preliminary clinical experience with genetic engineering of human vein grafts: Evidence for target gene inhibition. *Circulation* 96:14, 1997.

22. Mann MJ, Gibbons GH, Kernoff RS, et al: Genetic engineering of vein grafts resistant to atherosclerosis. *Proc Natl Acad Sci USA* 92:4502–4506, 1995.

23. Isner JM, Walsh K, Rosenfield K, et al: Clinical protocol: Arterial gene therapy for restenosis. *Hum Gene Ther* 7:989–1011, 1996.

24. DeYoung MB, Dichek DA: Gene therapy for restenosis. Are we ready? *Circ Res* 82:306–313, 1998.

25. Isner JM, Walsh K, Symes JF, et al: Arterial gene therapy for therapeutic angiogenesis in patients with peripheral artery disease. *Circulation* 91:2687-2692, 1995.

Index

269